THE A.G.E. FOOD GUIDE

A QUICK R
AND THE A

HELEN VLASSARA, MD
SANDRA WOODRUFF, MS, RD

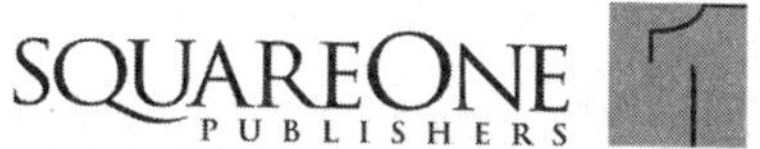

The information and advice contained in this book are based upon the research and the personal and professional experiences of the authors. They are not intended as a substitute for consulting with a healthcare professional. The publisher and authors are not responsible for any adverse effects or consequences resulting from the use of any of the suggestions, preparations, or procedures discussed in this book. All matters pertaining to your physical health should be supervised by a healthcare professional who can provide medical care tailored to meet individual needs.

COVER DESIGNER: Jeannie Tudor
TYPESETTER: Gary A. Rosenberg
IN-HOUSE EDITORS: Marie Caratozzolo and Joanne Abrams

Square One Publishers
115 Herricks Road • Garden City Park, NY 11040
516-535-2010 • 877-900-BOOK
www.SquareOnePublishers.com

ISBN: 978-0-7570-0429-2 (pb)
978-0-7570-5429-7 (eb)

Copyright © 2017 by Helen Vlassara and Sandra Woodruff

All rights reserved. No part of this publication may be reproduced, scanned, uploaded, stored in a retrieval system, or transmitted, in any form or by any means, electronic, mechanical, photocopying, recording, or otherwise, without the prior written permission of the publisher.

Printed in the United States of America

10 9 8 7 6 5 4 3 2 1

CONTENTS

PART TWO

INTRODUCTION

When Dr. Helen Vlassara and researchers at The Rockefeller University of New York began conducting studies on diabetes and its effects on the body, they focused on a fascinating group of complex substances that accumulate in the tissues. What they didn't know was that they were on their way to making some revolutionary discoveries. Over time, the compounds they explored—called *advanced glycation end products,* or *AGEs*—were found to be a cause of not just the devastating complications of diabetes, but also of diabetes itself. Subsequently, these toxic substances were linked to a wide range of other serious conditions, including cardiovascular disease, kidney disease, Alzheimer's disease, obesity, bone and joint problems, and other so-called diseases of aging. Moreover, they learned that most of these compounds enter the human body through the foods that people eat. The more AGEs people consume, the greater the likelihood of harm.

Once the team discovered the undeniable links between high AGE levels in the body, chronic disease, and a diet high in AGEs, they were faced with several questions. How do you count the AGEs in food? Which foods are highest in AGEs, and which foods are lowest? Dr. Vlassara and her colleagues had no option but to take up the task of determining the AGE levels of hundreds of foods. It took over ten years to develop new tools to bridge the gaps in their knowledge. Hundreds of thousands of tests later, they published the AGE levels of a wide range of foods and beverages.

Based on years of research and testing, this book is an easy-to-use guide to the AGE levels in food. Whether you are trying to avoid or manage a medical condition or you simply want to maintain good health, you're sure to find it invaluable as you learn about AGEs and use the guide to make smart food choices.

The book begins by answering a number of important questions about AGEs. Here, you'll get a crash course in AGEs—what they are and how they are associated with many conditions. As you already know, the chief source of these toxic substances is the foods you eat, and you'll learn how to choose and prepare foods in a way that reduces your consumption of AGEs. The fact is that you don't have to give up the foods you love to lower AGEs and experience greater health. By properly balancing high-AGE choices with low-AGE choices and preparing your foods using simple AGE-less cooking techniques, you can enjoy health-promoting meals that are both delicious and satisfying. In fact, a low-AGE diet has many similarities with the

Mediterranean diet, which is renowned for both its fine cuisine and its many health benefits.

After the Q and A section, you'll find the heart of the book: The AGE food guide, which includes two tables. The first table presents an alphabetical listing of hundreds of common foods and beverages, along with their AGE levels. Here, you can quickly find each food under its name, such as "Cheddar cheese," "Whole wheat bread," or "Salmon." The second table presents foods under logical categories such as "Cheeses," "Breads," and "Fish/Seafood." When you use this table, you'll be able to see the AGE levels of a variety of choices in a given category. For instance, by searching "Cheeses," you'll soon discover that lower-fat Cheddar cheese provides fewer AGEs than full-fat Cheddar, making the lower-fat product a wiser option for a low-AGE diet. Because cooking methods make such a big difference in the AGE levels of certain ingredients, listings of foods like chicken, beef, and eggs include the AGE levels for dishes cooked several different ways. For example, under "Chicken," you'll be able to quickly see that poached chicken is far lower in AGEs than grilled or fried chicken, making poaching a healthier choice. You'll also find that instead of stating specific numbers of AGE kilounits—numbers that can be affected by even small differences in food samplings—this guide identifies the AGE *range* for each food as being Very Low, Low, Medium, High, Very High, or Highest. This allows you to immediately understand the food's level of AGEs so that you can evaluate its suitability for your diet. Meanwhile, intriguing tips have been sprinkled throughout the guide, helping you make the best food choices possible.

We believe that what Dr. Vlassara and her team learned about AGEs and their profound negative effects on health and aging is one of the most exciting discoveries of the twenty-first century. Not only did their research identify an important contributor to disease, but it empowered each of us to take control of our own well-being by making simple changes in the way we select and cook our foods. This guide was designed to help you every step of the way. Turn the page, and learn how *The AGE Food Guide* can change your life.

PART ONE

FREQUENTLY ASKED QUESTIONS ABOUT AGEs

This book is an easy-to-use guide to the AGE (advanced glycation end product) levels of various common foods and beverages. Whether you are interested in avoiding or managing a specific disorder, such as diabetes or cardiovascular disease, or you want to simply improve your overall well-being, the table that begins on page 28 will help you do so. But if the concept of AGEs is a new one for you, it makes sense to take a little time to learn about it. That's why this simple question-and-answer section was written. It will first introduce you to AGEs and explain the types of damage that these common compounds can cause in the body. It will then explain the relationship of AGEs to food and help you understand how by avoiding excess AGEs in your diet, you can safeguard your health.

AGE BASICS

What are AGEs?

AGEs, or *advanced glycation end products,* are compounds that are produced when proteins or certain types of fats (lipids) react with sugars. It all starts when a sugar molecule latches onto a protein or fat in a process known as *glycation.* The newly glycated compound then goes through a series of changes to ultimately form an advanced glycation end product. In other words, AGEs can be viewed as modified proteins or fats. As such, their structure and function in the body can become altered, and they are no longer "normal." Due to their often toxic properties, AGEs are sometimes referred to as *glycotoxins.* And since they act as oxidants, AGEs are also known as *glycoxidants.*

While AGEs can be produced inside the body, from our own sugars and proteins or fats, most AGEs come from outside the body, in our foods. There are literally hundreds of different types of AGEs, some of which are tied to chronic disease and premature aging. This book lists the food levels of a common AGE compound that is used as a "representative" AGE because it has been linked to many health problems.

How do AGEs harm the body?

As discussed above, AGEs are modified ("abnormal") proteins and lipids, many of which are toxic substances. AGEs can harm the body in several distinct ways. For instance, AGEs are seen by the body as "irritants," so they provoke the immune system, triggering chronic systemic inflammation. This type of inflammation is well known as an underlying cause of many chronic diseases. (See page 11 to learn more about inflammation.) As oxidants, AGEs also damage the body's tissues in much the way that acid rusts metal. And acting like glue, AGEs bind proteins together in a process known as *cross-linking*. This explains why joints, muscles, and tendons become stiff as we get older. This also explains the "hardening of the arteries" that comes with age. In addition, AGEs are known to suppress vital "host defenses" in the body. These protectors, with names such as SIRT1 and AGER1, help keep us well by quenching inflammation, neutralizing free radicals, and performing many other essential tasks. The changes that are brought on by AGEs can ultimately cause the cells and organs of the body to malfunction.

Understanding the various ways in which AGEs cause harm makes it easy to see how they can cause so many seemingly different diseases. For example, excess AGEs can bring about insulin resistance, help retain body fat in the form of harmful AGE-fat, hasten the wrinkling and other skin changes that come with age, and cause cataracts. They have even been found to damage cells of the brain. In fact, AGEs cause problems in seemingly inexhaustible ways.

AGEs AND CHRONIC DISEASE

How are AGEs associated with diabetes?

Diabetes is a disorder marked by high levels of sugar (glucose) in the blood. It occurs when the body either doesn't produce enough *insulin*—the hormone that enables glucose to be used for energy by the body—or doesn't respond properly to insulin.

AGEs and diabetes appear to be related on many levels. First, by damaging the insulin-producing cells of the pancreas, causing chronic inflammation, and producing other changes in the body, high AGE levels appear to promote the development of diabetes. Then, because in diabetes, more sugar is available to interact with proteins and lipids, this disorder can significantly increase the formation of AGEs in the body. In fact, studies in people with diabetes were what provided the first clues about AGEs and their destructive nature. A large body of research has shown that AGEs are involved in and even drive the most devastating complications of diabetes, including cardiovascular disease and kidney disease. Eventually, the evidence came full-circle and demonstrated that in the relative absence of AGEs, these complications are slowed down or do not develop at all—despite the presence of high blood sugar levels. So AGEs promote the development of diabetes, and once diabetes occurs, these substances can create further serious complications.

How are AGEs associated with cardiovascular disease?

The term *cardiovascular disease* refers to a variety of disorders that affect the heart and/or blood vessels. Included among these disorders are blood vessel diseases such as coronary artery disease, heart failure, and stroke.

AGEs are strongly associated with common blood vessel and heart problems. As these dangerous compounds build up with time, they "weld" proteins together, making blood vessels progressively thicker and inflexible. When stiff blood vessels cannot dilate (open), the result is called *arteriosclerosis* (hardening of the arteries), which leads to high blood pressure and heart disease. AGEs also cause blood vessel rigidity by reducing the activity of nitric oxide, a powerful compound that normally widens the blood vessels so they can carry more blood to the tissues. In addition, AGEs cause small blood vessels (capillaries) to become leaky; encourage the formation of blood clots that block blood vessels, potentially leading to stroke; oxidize LDL (bad) cholesterol so that it is harder to remove from the blood; and oxidize HDL (good) cholesterol so that it no longer has a protective function.

How are AGEs associated with dementia?

Dementia is a chronic disorder marked by problems with memory, the ability to concentrate, and the ability to learn. There are many causes of dementia, but most often, dementia develops over many years, with the gradual erosion of cognitive function caused either by injury to the brain itself, as in Alzheimer's disease, or by impaired blood flow to the brain, as in vascular dementia.

It is well established that regardless of its cause, dementia is strongly linked to chronic inflammation and oxidant stress, and high levels of AGEs inside the body are key drivers of both. AGEs can contribute to brain disease in a variety of other ways, as well. By causing blood vessels to become leaky, AGEs can damage the protective barrier that insulates the brain from the rest of the body. This, in turn, allows AGEs to get inside the brain, where they can promote inflammation, leading to brain injury. There is also convincing evidence that AGEs can trigger or accelerate the formation of *amyloid plaques* and *neurofibrillary tangles* (or *tau tangles*), brain-damaging structures that are hallmarks of Alzheimer's disease.

How are AGEs associated with kidney disease?

The kidneys are the body's main "exit" for excreting toxic AGEs, and therefore, as long as they function normally, they constantly protect our health. A decline in kidney function—a closing down of this important exit—raises AGE levels in the blood and sets the stage for widespread trouble, including greater damage to the kidneys and all other organs.

This may be why kidney disease is linked to diabetes, heart disease, cancer, Alzheimer's disease, and aging.

Evidence supports the idea that kidney disease favors a buildup of body AGEs and that an increase in body AGEs can lead to further decline in kidney function, perpetuating a cycle of disease and destruction. Fortunately, studies have shown that patients with chronic kidney disease who are treated with a low-AGE diet for a few weeks experience a remarkable decrease in circulating AGEs as well as in levels of markers of inflammation and oxidative stress.

How are AGEs associated with chronic inflammation?

The body has a built-in mechanism to defend itself against threats such as bacteria, damaged cells and tissues, and foreign substances. This process, known as the *inflammatory response,* is necessary for health and survival. Immune cells such as white blood cells swarm the injured area, attack and destroy the offenders, and clean up the mess to get tissues ready for repair and renewal. When the threat has been removed—usually within a few hours or a few days—inflammation ends, and the body is able to heal. This short-term response is known as *acute inflammation.*

If the body continues to be exposed to irritants, however, a persistent low-grade form of inflammation can develop. This condition is known as *chronic inflammation.* Food AGEs, which constantly flow into the body, provide an abundant source of irritants that can drive and maintain chronic inflammation. As AGEs begin to pile up in tissues, the immune system sets out to destroy them, and in the process, it may inadvertently damage some of the surrounding tissues. The more AGEs there are, the greater this "collateral damage." Over time, the tissues become so injured that organs begin to malfunction, leading to chronic disease. In fact, low-grade, chronic inflammation has been linked to a host of health problems, including cardiovascular disease, diabetes, kidney disease, dementia, and many other conditions that are common in aging. In studies of people with chronic inflammation, the extent of inflammation has been found to be proportional to the level of AGEs in the body.

How are AGEs associated with overweight and obesity?

Overweight or *obesity,* both of which refer to having an excess amount of body fat, affect the majority of adults and alarming numbers of children in modern society.

Excess body fat is believed to be associated with AGEs in a number of ways. For one thing, AGEs add enticing flavor, aroma, and color to foods, and this drives us to overeat. As you will learn later, some foods are higher in AGEs than others, and for most people, high-AGE foods such as steak, pizza, and fried chicken are the most inviting. When we eat more calories than we burn for energy, the excess calories are deposited in the body as fat and, therefore, as extra weight.

Studies also suggest that AGEs may contribute to obesity by favoring the accumulation of AGE-rich visceral fat, or belly fat, which can be extremely difficult—even impossible—to eliminate. AGEs may favor fat storage by suppressing certain protective mechanisms, such as SIRT1, which is crucial for moving fatty acids from visceral fat out to the liver to be metabolized. Most important, AGE-belly fat is known to spew out inflammatory substances into the bloodstream, causing the widespread chronic inflammation discussed earlier.

What other health disorders are associated with AGEs?

By virtue of their ability to ramp up inflammation, cross-link proteins, damage tissues and organs, and suppress the body's host defenses, AGEs can cause the body to malfunction in a wide variety of ways, only a few of which were discussed above. Additional disorders that appear to be associated with AGEs include:

- ❑ Arthritis
- ❑ Intervertebral disc disease
- ❑ Muscle changes and muscle loss
- ❑ Osteoporosis (bone fragility)
- ❑ Skin problems such as loss of elasticity and cellulite

- ❏ Vision problems such as cataracts
- ❏ Wound healing problems

AGEs AND FOOD

Where do most of the body's AGEs come from?

On page 6, you learned that AGEs can be produced both inside the body from our own sugars and proteins or fats, and outside the body from the sugars, proteins, and fats that are present in our foods. For a long time, it was believed that we don't absorb AGEs from food, and that any AGEs found in the body were created in the body. Studies eventually proved this to be untrue. Although the body continually produces some AGEs, *most AGEs come from outside the body through the diet.*

It's important to remember that the kidneys perform the task of flushing AGEs out of the body, just as they flush out other harmful substances. But the kidneys have a limited ability to eliminate AGEs. When these hard-working organs are healthy, a "reasonable" amount of AGEs can be removed. But when kidney function is decreased or too many AGEs are consumed through foods, a surplus of AGEs slowly disperses throughout the tissues, creating havoc.

Can a low-AGE diet improve your health?

You now know that high levels of AGEs can cause a host of problems. The good news is that since most of the AGEs in the body come from foods, you can lower your AGE levels and improve your health by eating a low-AGE diet.

Studies in animals and humans indicate that reducing dietary AGEs to a safe level can help to lower chronic inflammation; protect vascular function (blood flow); help maintain normal brain function, including memory; lower the risk of developing diabetes; help normalize insulin resistance and reduce complications in people who already have diabetes; help prevent kidney disease; help prevent unwanted weight gain; help preserve the health of the spine; and enhance health in many other ways.

How low do dietary AGEs have to go to protect health? Our studies have shown that a safe intake is below 8,000 AGE kilounits per day—about half of the AGEs found in most adult diets. Moreover, on a low-AGE diet, improvements—indicated by lower levels of inflammation and improved host defenses—can be seen within just a few weeks.

It is important to understand that in addition to helping prevent serious health problems, a lower-AGE diet may actually *reverse* existing conditions. Evidence shows that a low-AGE diet can improve diabetes by reversing insulin resistance—a serious problem in many people who already have diabetes—and can improve faulty vascular (blood vessel) and kidney function by reducing chronic inflammation. So it is never too late to start a low-AGE diet.

Which foods are generally highest in AGEs?

Meat typically adds more AGEs to the diet than any other food group. Beef tends to have the highest levels of AGEs, followed by poultry and pork. Fish has more moderate AGE levels, while eggs and legumes (dried beans, peas, and lentils)—which can be eaten in place of meats—rank lowest on the AGE scale for proteins. Leaner cuts of meat have fewer AGEs than fattier cuts, but even lean red meats and skinless chicken can provide high levels of AGEs when cooked with high-dry heat. (You'll learn more about how cooking affects the AGE levels in foods on page 17.) Other foods that are especially high in AGEs are cheeses and fats.

Which foods are generally lowest in AGEs?

Plant foods—which include vegetables, fruits, whole grains, and legumes—contain lower amounts of AGEs than animal foods. Vegetables and fruits are naturally very low in AGEs owing to their relatively low content of protein and fat and their high content of water. The high amounts of antioxidants and vitamins in vegetables and fruits may also diminish AGE formation in these foods. Freezing, canning, and juicing do not raise AGE content. Drying—used to turn grapes into raisins, for instance—does raise AGE levels. However, the amount of AGEs in dried fruit is very small compared with AGE levels in meats, cheeses, and fats. Moreover, both starchy vegetables (such as corn and potatoes) and non-starchy vegetables (such as green beans and carrots) are low in AGEs.

As you'll learn below, dry-heat cooking methods such as grilling, broiling, and roasting can greatly raise the AGE content of all foods, including fruits and vegetables. But even when prepared using these techniques, plant foods have just a small fraction of the AGEs found in grilled or broiled meats.

CONTROLLING AGEs

How does cooking affect the AGE level in foods?

All foods naturally contain some AGEs, even in their uncooked state. Cooking causes additional AGEs to form, but this does not mean that you must consume all of your food raw. By choosing the right cooking methods, you can greatly minimize the formation of new AGEs.

The main cause for the increase of AGEs during cooking is high-dry heat, which is present when you grill, roast, bake, broil, or fry foods. Any kind of cooking that uses a lot of heat, chars the outside of the food, and dries out the food causes a dramatic rise in toxic AGEs. That's why browning, one of the hallmarks of high-dry heat cooking, is a sure sign that AGE formation has taken place. On the other hand, moist-heat cooking methods—such as poaching, steaming, stewing, and braising

—minimize the formation of further AGEs. It is important to note that some foods, such as oils and cheeses, which don't have the classic "browned" appearance of roasted or grilled foods, can also deliver large amounts of AGEs. This is due to the fact that many AGE compounds lack the typical gold-brown color.

To appreciate the effect that different cooking methods have on AGE counts, consider that chicken which is roasted (a dry-heat cooking method) can have more than five times as many AGEs as chicken which is poached (a moist-heat cooking method). Deep-fried chicken, which adds a large amount of oil to the mix, creates an even more extreme rise in AGEs. The table that begins on page 28 will show you the effect that different cooking methods have on the AGE levels of various foods.

How does commercial processing affect the AGE level in foods?

We've already mentioned that AGEs add color, flavor, and aroma to food. Most people become conditioned to prefer the appearance, taste, and smell of higher-AGE foods rather than lower-AGE foods. The food industry understands that AGEs are commercially valuable, and that foods may sell better—and be eaten in larger quantities—when they contain lots of AGEs. To cater to the public's tastes, numerous products are made with high-heat processing. Consider all the grain products, such as crackers and chips, that are fried in oil or heat-processed until they are dry and crisp. Chemicals are also used to mimic the flavors that we love, and many of these additives are chemically synthesized AGEs. For these reasons, commercially processed foods can be a significant source of AGEs.

This doesn't mean that all processed foods are bad. Plant-based products such as rolled oats, whole grain pasta, frozen vegetables, and canned beans are convenient, high in nutrients, and very appropriate for an AGE-less diet. The table that begins on page 28 provides specific information about the AGE levels in various processed foods.

What is the connection between sugar and AGEs?

You have already learned that sugar plays a principal role in the formation of AGEs (see page 6). When sugar or other high-sugar sweeteners such as honey are added to foods and heated—which occurs in the making of cookies, for instance—the sugar can react with fats and proteins to make AGEs. That's why even though sugar and other sweeteners are relatively low in AGEs, you should limit their use as much as possible. It's worth noting, too, that a diet high in refined and processed carbohydrates can contribute to obesity, insulin resistance, and eventually, diabetes.

Does portion size matter?

When you are following a low-AGE diet, portion size definitely matters. The AGE count ranges stated in the tables in this book are for specific portion sizes—one ounce of nuts or three ounces of chicken, for instance. If your serving size is larger, you will consume more AGEs. In fact, some people consume too many AGEs simply because they eat too much food—especially high-AGE foods such as grilled meats.

This doesn't mean that you will be hungry on a healthy low-AGE diet. It simply means that you should have generous portions of low-AGE foods such as vegetables and smaller portions of high-AGE foods such as meat.

What strategies can you use to lower the AGEs in your diet?

Because plant foods, such as vegetables and fruits, are lowest in AGEs, and animal foods, such as meat and cheese, are highest in AGEs, it's important to remember that at least three-quarters of your AGE-less diet should be comprised of plant foods. For this reason, you should be sure to include plenty of side dishes (vegetables, whole grains, and legumes) and salads in your diet. Following this guideline alone will help you limit AGEs by limiting your consumption of high-AGE foods.

It's worth noting that many lower-AGE foods are just plain healthier than higher-AGE foods. Think about fresh fruits and vegetables, beans, peas, and whole grains. These are the foods that provide an abundance of fiber, vitamins, and minerals, as well as beneficial compounds such as phytochemicals and antioxidants. These are also the foods that contribute to healthy body weight by preventing the storage of AGE-fat. It just makes sense to select those foods that are low in AGEs as often as possible.

Of course, as you've learned, the way you cook your foods will also have a significant effect on the amount of AGEs you consume with your meals. That's why, especially when cooking beef, chicken, and other high-AGE choices, you'll want to use moist-heat cooking methods such as stewing, braising, steaming, simmering, and poaching.

The table that begins on page 28 will help you home in on both the foods and the cooking methods that are most appropriate for a low-AGE diet. Remember, though, that you don't want to carry your diet to extremes and choose only low-AGE foods at the expense of good nutrition. By selecting a higher proportion of foods low in AGEs; limiting portions of high-AGE foods; avoiding low-nutrient processed foods, such as potato chips and cookies; and using AGE-less cooking techniques; you can create a satisfying well-balanced diet that will lower your risk of developing chronic disease while enhancing your well-being for years to come.

CONCLUSION

We believe that our research into AGEs—which took place over a period of decades—enabled us to identify a key reason why the body can malfunction, experience accelerated aging, and develop chronic disease. Perhaps most important, our research showed us how the toxic compounds known as AGEs can be controlled through the careful selection and preparation of foods.

This book is a guide to the AGEs in foods. It gives you the power to make smart dietary choices that can help you maintain or even restore your health. If you want to learn more about AGEs—their history and their science, as well as details of a low-AGE diet—read *Dr. Vlassara's AGE-Less Diet.*

HOW TO USE THIS GUIDE

The following tables in Part Two provide the AGE levels of common foods and beverages. The table that begins on page 28 presents an alphabetical listing of foods, while the table that starts on page 114 lists foods under common categories such as "Beverages," "Breads," "Cheeses," "Meats," etc. The table of category entries not only offers you a different way to look foods up, but also enables you to compare the AGE levels of foods within a group so that you can make healthy low-AGE choices.

For each food listed, the table first provides the portion size and then tells you whether the AGE level is Very Low (under 100 kU per serving), Low (between 100 and 500 kU per serving), Medium (between 501 and 1,000 kU per serving), High (between 1,001 and 3,000 kU per serving), Very High (between 3,001 and 5,000 kU per serving), or Highest (over 5,001 kU per serving). One kU, or kilounit, refers to one thousand AGE units in a standard amount of protein or lipid (fat). Although the term kilounit may be unfamiliar to you, you will quickly understand that this standard measurement allows us to compare the AGEs provided by different foods. The more kilounits there are, the more AGEs the food contains.

In the case of some foods, such as oven-braised turkey breast, two boxes—"Medium" and "High," for instance—have been marked. This indicates that the food is on the "borderline" of two categories, and therefore may belong in either category. A number of variables—such as the fat content of the turkey breast, the temperature of your oven, or the amount of time the food is cooked—can have an effect on the number of AGEs found in the final dish. This can push a food out of one category and into another.

You'll see that when a food can be cooked in different ways, the AGEs are listed for some of the most common methods used—poaching, steaming, broiling, boiling, roasting, etc. This information was included because the cooking method you choose can make a significant difference in the final AGE count. (See page 14 to learn more about this.) If you look up chicken, for instance, you'll find that while poached chicken breast is a medium AGE food, roasted chicken breast can be very high or even highest in AGEs, depending on whether the skin is removed. (Including the skin will increase the level of AGEs.) These listings will let you know how your cooking technique will affect the AGE count of your dish. Tips sprinkled throughout the tables will not only help you make wise food choices but also guide you in preparing foods in a way that minimizes AGE formation.

Remember that portion size does count. The AGE ranges stated in the tables in this book are for specific serving sizes—eight ounces of milk, one ounce of crackers, or three ounces of chicken, for instance. If your serving size is larger, you will boost your consumption of AGEs.

Since higher amounts of AGEs mean a higher risk of certain health problems (see page 8), you may be tempted to choose only low-AGE foods. Instead of an extreme low-AGE diet, however, we suggest that at least three-quarters of your AGE-less diet should be comprised of plant foods—fruits, vegetables, whole grains, and legumes. This will not only help limit your consumption of AGEs, but also make sure that you get all the nutrients you need for good health.

PART TWO

A-TO-Z LISTING OF BASIC FOODS

FOOD	Portion Size	Very Low 100 kU or less	Low 100–500 kU	Medium 501–1,000 kU	High 1,001–3,000 kU	Very High 3,001–5,000 kU	Highest 5,000–12,000 kU
Acai berries	3.5 oz	■					
Acorn squash							
baked	3.5 oz	■	■				
boiled	3.5 oz	■					
broiled	3.5 oz	■	■				
grilled	3.5 oz	■	■				
raw	3.5 oz	■					
roasted	3.5 oz	■	■				
steamed	3.5 oz	■					
Almonds							
raw	1 oz				■		
roasted	1 oz				■		
Amaranth	3.5 oz	■					

TIP

Avoid cheese with labels like "processed cheese," "prepared cheese product," or "cheese food." These foods have undergone additional heating, melting, and processing steps that raise their AGE content.

FOOD	Portion Size	Very Low 100 kU or less	Low 100–500 kU	Medium 501–1,000 kU	High 1,001–3,000 kU	Very High 3,001–5,000 kU	Highest 5,000–12,000 kU
American cheese							
low-fat	1 oz			■	■		
regular	1 oz				■		
Angel food cake	1 oz	■					
Apple							
baked	3.5 oz	■	■				

FOOD	Portion Size	Very Low 100 kU or less	Low 100–500 kU	Medium 501–1,000 kU	High 1,001–3,000 kU	Very High 3,001–5,000 kU	Highest 5,000–12,000 kU
raw	3.5 oz	■					
simmered	3.5 oz	■					
Apple cider vinegar	1 Tbs	■					
Apple Crumb Pie, Dutch (Mrs. Smith's)	1/8 pie			■			
Apple juice	8 oz	■					
Apple pie (McDonald's)	1 pie			■			
Apple Pie, Dutch Crumb (Mrs. Smith's)	1/8 pie			■			
Apricot							
baked	3.5 oz	■	■				
grilled	3.5 oz	■	■				
poached	3.5 oz	■					
raw	3.5 oz	■					
Arborio rice	3.5 oz	■					
Arugula (rocket)	3.5 oz	■					
Asparagus							
boiled	3.5 oz	■					
broiled	3.5 oz	■	■				
grilled	3.5 oz	■	■				
raw	3.5 oz	■					
roasted	3.5 oz	■	■				
sautéed w/cooking spray	3.5 oz	■	■				
steamed	3.5 oz	■					

FOOD	Portion Size	Very Low 100 kU or less	Low 100–500 kU	Medium 501–1,000 kU	High 1,001–3,000 kU	Very High 3,001–5,000 kU	Highest 5,000–12,000 kU
stir-fried w/cooking spray	3.5 oz	■	■				
Aspartame, sugar substitute	1 tsp	■					
Aubergine (eggplant)							
broiled	3.5 oz	■	■				
grilled	3.5 oz	■	■				
raw	3.5 oz	■					
roasted	3.5 oz	■	■				
sautéed w/cooking spray	3.5 oz	■	■				
steamed	3.5 oz	■					
stewed	3.5 oz	■					
stir-fried w/cooking spray	3.5 oz	■	■				
Avocado	1 oz		■				
Baby bella mushrooms (crimini)							
baked	3.5 oz	■	■				
boiled	3.5 oz	■					
broiled	3.5 oz	■	■				
grilled	3.5 oz	■	■				
raw	3.5 oz	■					
roasted	3.5 oz	■	■				
sautéed w/cooking spray	3.5 oz	■	■				
steamed	3.5 oz	■					
stir-fried w/cooking spray	3.5 oz	■	■				

FOOD	Portion Size	Very Low 100 kU or less	Low 100–500 kU	Medium 501–1,000 kU	High 1,001–3,000 kU	Very High 3,001–5,000 kU	Highest 5,000–12,000 kU
Bacon							
microwaved	2 slices				■		
pan-fried	2 slices						■
Bacon, egg & cheese biscuit (fast food)	1 sandwich					■	
Bacon, vegetarian, microwaved	2 slices		■				
Bacon bits, imitation (soy)	0.5 oz		■				
Bagel							
toasted	2 oz		■				
untoasted	2 oz	■					
Balsamic vinegar	1 Tbs	■					
Banana							
baked	3.5 oz	■	■				
grilled	3.5 oz	■	■				
pan-fried w/cooking spray	3.5 oz	■	■				
raw	3.5 oz	■					
Banana bread, low-fat	2 oz	■	■				
Bar, snack							
Granola, Chocolate Chunk (Quaker)	1 bar		■				
Granola, Peanut Butter/Chocolate Chip (Quaker)	1 bar			■			
Nutrigrain, Apple Cinnamon	1 bar			■			

FOOD	Portion Size	Very Low 100 kU or less	Low 100–500 kU	Medium 501–1,000 kU	High 1,001–3,000 kU	Very High 3,001–5,000 kU	Highest 5,000–12,000 kU
Rice Krispies Treat	1 bar		■	■			
Barley	3.5 oz	■					
Basmati rice	3.5 oz	■					
Beans, black							
boiled	3.5 oz		■				
canned, unheated	3.5 oz		■				
raw	3.5 oz	■	■				
Beans, cannellini							
boiled	3.5 oz		■				
canned, unheated	3.5 oz		■				
raw	3.5 oz	■	■				
Beans, fava							
boiled	3.5 oz		■				
raw	3.5 oz	■	■				
Beans, Great Northern							
boiled	3.5 oz		■				
canned, unheated	3.5 oz		■				
raw	3.5 oz	■	■				
Beans, green							
baked	3.5 oz	■	■				
boiled	3.5 oz	■					
canned, unheated	3.5 oz	■					
raw	3.5 oz	■					
sautéed w/cooking spray	3.5 oz	■	■				

FOOD	Portion Size	Very Low 100 kU or less	Low 100–500 kU	Medium 501–1,000 kU	High 1,001–3,000 kU	Very High 3,001–5,000 kU	Highest 5,000–12,000 kU
steamed	3.5 oz	■					
stir-fried w/cooking spray	3.5 oz	■	■				
Beans, kidney, red							
boiled	3.5 oz		■				
canned, unheated	3.5 oz		■				
raw	3.5 oz	■	■				
Beans, lima							
boiled	3.5 oz		■				
canned, unheated	3.5 oz		■				
raw	3.5 oz	■	■				
Beans, navy							
boiled	3.5 oz		■				
canned, unheated	3.5 oz		■				
raw	3.5 oz	■	■				
Beans, pink							
boiled	3.5 oz		■				
canned, unheated	3.5 oz		■				
raw	3.5 oz	■	■				
Beans, pinto							
boiled	3.5 oz		■				
canned, unheated	3.5 oz		■				
raw	3.5 oz	■	■				
Beans/Legumes. ***See*** **individual varieties.**							
Beef, corned, low-fat	3 oz			■			

FOOD	Portion Size	Very Low 100 kU or less	Low 100–500 kU	Medium 501–1,000 kU	High 1,001–3,000 kU	Very High 3,001–5,000 kU	Highest 5,000–12,000 kU
Beef, ground							
80% lean, pan-browned	3 oz					■	
91% lean, grass-fed, pan-browned	3 oz			■			
91% lean, grass-fed, raw	3 oz		■				
93% lean, pan-browned	3 oz			■	■		
93% lean, raw	3 oz			■			
Beef, raw	3 oz			■			
Beef, roast	3 oz						■

TIP

When buying beef, choose organic grass-fed products whenever possible. Meat from grass-fed animals is lower in AGEs than meat from conventionally raised animals.

FOOD	Portion Size	Very Low	Low	Medium	High	Very High	Highest
Beef, shoulder cut							
raw	3 oz			■			
stewed	3 oz				■		
Beef, top round chunks							
raw	3 oz		■	■			
stewed	3 oz			■			
Beef, top round roast							
oven-braised	3 oz				■		
pressure-cooked	3 oz				■		
raw	3 oz		■	■			
Beef bologna	3 oz				■		

FOOD	Portion Size	Very Low 100 kU or less	Low 100–500 kU	Medium 501–1,000 kU	High 1,001–3,000 kU	Very High 3,001–5,000 kU	Highest 5,000–12,000 kU
Beef bouillon	1 cup	■					
Beef frankfurter							
boiled	3 oz					■	■
broiled	3 oz						■
Beef hamburger patty (fast food)	3 oz					■	
Beef hamburger patty, 93% lean							
grilled (nonstick grill)	3 oz				■		
pan-cooked	3 oz				■		
Beef meatball							
simmered in broth	3 oz					■	
93% lean, simmered in tomato sauce	3 oz				■		
Beef meatloaf							
oven-baked	3 oz				■		
93% lean, oven-baked	3 oz			■			
Beef salami, kosher	3 oz			■			
Beef steak							
broiled	3 oz						■
grilled (nonstick grill)	3 oz						■
microwaved	3 oz				■		
pan-fried	3 oz						■
raw	3 oz			■			
stir-fried (strips)	3 oz						■

FOOD	Portion Size	Very Low 100 kU or less	Low 100–500 kU	Medium 501–1,000 kU	High 1,001–3,000 kU	Very High 3,001–5,000 kU	Highest 5,000–12,000 kU
Beef steak, top sirloin, trimmed							
grilled (nonstick grill), rare	3 oz			■			
grilled (nonstick grill), medium	3 oz				■		
grilled (nonstick grill), well done	3 oz				■		
raw	3 oz		■	■			
Beer	9 oz	■					
Beet (beetroot)							
boiled	3.5 oz	■					
raw	3.5 oz	■					
roasted	3.5 oz	■	■				
steamed	3.5 oz	■					
Beetroot (beet)							
boiled	3.5 oz	■					
raw	3.5 oz	■					
roasted	3.5 oz	■	■				
steamed	3.5 oz	■					
Belgian endive (endive, witloof)	3.5 oz	■					
Bell pepper							
grilled	3.5 oz	■	■				
raw	3.5 oz	■					
roasted	3.5 oz	■	■				

FOOD	Portion Size	Very Low 100 kU or less	Low 100–500 kU	Medium 501–1,000 kU	High 1,001–3,000 kU	Very High 3,001–5,000 kU	Highest 5,000–12,000 kU
sautéed w/cooking spray	3.5 oz	■	■				
steamed	3.5 oz	■					
stir-fried w/cooking spray	3.5 oz	■	■				
Beverages. ***See*** **individual varieties.**							
Bibb lettuce	3.5 oz	■					
Biscotti cookie, vanilla almond	1 oz			■			
Biscuit	2 oz			■			
Biscuit, bacon, egg & cheese (fast food)	1 sandwich					■	
Black beans							
boiled	3.5 oz		■				
canned, unheated	3.5 oz		■				
raw	3.5 oz	■	■				
Black forbidden rice, Chinese	3.5 oz	■					
Black japonica rice	3.5 oz	■					
Black-eyed peas							
boiled	3.5 oz		■				
canned, unheated	3.5 oz		■				
raw	3.5 oz	■	■				
Blackberries							
cooked	3.5 oz	■					
raw	3.5 oz	■					

FOOD	Portion Size	Very Low 100 kU or less	Low 100–500 kU	Medium 501–1,000 kU	High 1,001–3,000 kU	Very High 3,001–5,000 kU	Highest 5,000–12,000 kU
Blue cheese salad dressing	1 Tbs	■	■				
Blueberries							
cooked	3.5 oz	■					
raw	3.5 oz	■					
Boca Burger (soy)							
microwaved	1 burger	■					
oven-baked	1 burger	■	■				
pan-cooked w/cooking spray	1 burger	■					
pan-cooked w/olive oil	1 burger	■	■				
Bok choy							
boiled	3.5 oz	■					
broiled	3.5 oz	■	■				
grilled	3.5 oz	■	■				
raw	3.5 oz	■					
sautéed w/cooking spray	3.5 oz	■	■				
steamed	3.5 oz	■					
stir-fried w/cooking spray	3.5 oz	■	■				
Bologna, beef	3 oz				■		
Boston lettuce	3.5 oz	■					
Bouillon							
beef	1 cup	■					
chicken	1 cup	■					

FOOD	Portion Size	Very Low 100 kU or less	Low 100–500 kU	Medium 501–1,000 kU	High 1,001–3,000 kU	Very High 3,001–5,000 kU	Highest 5,000–12,000 kU
Bourbon whiskey	1.5 oz	■					
Boysenberries							
cooked	3.5 oz	■					
raw	3.5 oz	■					
Bran flakes cereal	1 cup	■					
Bran muffin	2.5 oz		■				
Bread							
Italian	2 oz	■					
Italian, toasted	2 oz	■					
pita	2 oz	■					
white	2 oz	■					
white, toasted	2 oz	■					
whole wheat	2 oz	■					
whole wheat, toasted	2 oz	■					
Bread, banana, low-fat	2 oz	■					
Breadsticks	1 oz	■					
Breast milk							
fresh	1 oz	■					
frozen	1 oz	■					

TIP

For maximum fiber and nutrients, choose whole grain breads. To keep AGEs low, avoid higher-fat choices such as biscuits and croissants, which provide more AGEs. Toast the bread if you like, but skip high-fat AGE-rich spreads such as cream cheese and butter.

FOOD	Portion Size	Very Low 100 kU or less	Low 100–500 kU	Medium 501–1,000 kU	High 1,001–3,000 kU	Very High 3,001–5,000 kU	Highest 5,000–12,000 kU
Brie cheese	1 oz				■		
Broccoli							
baked	3.5 oz	■	■				
boiled	3.5 oz	■					
broiled	3.5 oz	■	■				
grilled	3.5 oz	■	■				
raw	3.5 oz	■					
roasted	3.5 oz	■	■				
sautéed w/cooking spray	3.5 oz	■	■				
steamed	3.5 oz	■					
stir-fried w/cooking spray	3.5 oz	■	■				
Broccoli rabe (rapini)							
baked	3.5 oz	■	■				
boiled	3.5 oz	■					
raw	3.5 oz	■					
sautéed w/cooking spray	3.5 oz	■	■				
steamed	3.5 oz	■					
stir-fried w/cooking spray	3.5 oz	■	■				
Broccoli timbale	3.5 oz		■				
Broccolini							
baked	3.5 oz	■	■				
boiled	3.5 oz	■					
broiled	3.5 oz	■	■				
grilled	3.5 oz	■	■				

FOOD	Portion Size	Very Low 100 kU or less	Low 100–500 kU	Medium 501–1,000 kU	High 1,001–3,000 kU	Very High 3,001–5,000 kU	Highest 5,000–12,000 kU
raw	3.5 oz	■					
roasted	3.5 oz	■	■				
sautéed w/cooking spray	3.5 oz	■	■				
steamed	3.5 oz	■					
stir-fried w/cooking spray	3.5 oz	■	■				
Broth							
chicken	1 cup	■					
vegetable	1 cup	■					
Brown rice	3.5 oz	■					

TIP

Keep the amount of AGEs in vegetables low by going easy on added fats. A good tip is to add just a drizzle of extra-virgin olive oil instead of drenching your dish with oil, butter, or cheese sauce.

FOOD	Portion Size	Very Low	Low	Medium	High	Very High	Highest
Brussels sprouts							
baked	3.5 oz	■	■				
boiled	3.5 oz	■					
broiled	3.5 oz	■	■				
grilled	3.5 oz	■	■				
raw	3.5 oz	■					
roasted	3.5 oz	■	■				
sautéed w/cooking spray	3.5 oz	■	■				
steamed	3.5 oz	■					
stir-fried w/cooking spray	3.5 oz	■	■				

FOOD	Portion Size	Very Low 100 kU or less	Low 100–500 kU	Medium 501–1,000 kU	High 1,001–3,000 kU	Very High 3,001–5,000 kU	Highest 5,000–12,000 kU
Buckwheat	3.5 oz	■					
Burger, chicken, 89% lean							
pan-fried w/cooking spray	3 oz				■		
Burger, soy (Boca Burger)							
microwaved	1 burger	■					
oven-baked	1 burger	■	■				
pan-cooked w/cooking spray	1 burger	■					
pan-cooked w/olive oil	1 burger	■	■				
Burger, turkey							
broiled	3 oz					■	
pan-fried	3 oz						■
pan-fried, 94% lean	3 oz				■		
Burger, California Veggie (Amy's)							
microwaved	1 burger	■					
oven-baked	1 burger		■				
pan-cooked w/cooking spray	1 burger	■	■				
pan-cooked w/olive oil	1 burger		■				

TIP

When reheating foods, the microwave oven can be a good choice, as it tends to heat foods without drying them out. This will minimize the formation of new AGEs. For foods without liquid, add some broth, sauce, or gravy, and reheat just long enough to bring the food to the desired temperature.

FOOD	Portion Size	Very Low 100 kU or less	Low 100–500 kU	Medium 501–1,000 kU	High 1,001–3,000 kU	Very High 3,001–5,000 kU	Highest 5,000–12,000 kU
Butter							
browned	1 Tbs				■		
clarified	1 Tbs				■	■	
unsalted	1 Tbs				■		
whipped	1 Tbs				■		
Butter lettuce	3.5 oz	■					
Butternut squash							
baked	3.5 oz	■	■				
boiled	3.5 oz	■					
broiled	3.5 oz	■	■				
grilled	3.5 oz	■	■				
raw	3.5 oz	■					
roasted	3.5 oz	■	■				
steamed	3.5 oz	■					
Button mushrooms (white button)							
baked	3.5 oz	■	■				
boiled	3.5 oz	■					
broiled	3.5 oz	■	■				
grilled	3.5 oz	■	■				
raw	3.5 oz	■					
roasted	3.5 oz	■	■				
sautéed w/cooking spray	3.5 oz	■	■				
steamed	3.5 oz	■					
stir-fried w/cooking spray	3.5 oz	■	■				

FOOD	Portion Size	Very Low 100 kU or less	Low 100–500 kU	Medium 501–1,000 kU	High 1,001–3,000 kU	Very High 3,001–5,000 kU	Highest 5,000–12,000 kU
Cabbage							
boiled	3.5 oz	■					
raw	3.5 oz	■					
sautéed w/cooking spray	3.5 oz	■	■				
steamed	3.5 oz	■					
stir-fried w/cooking spray	3.5 oz	■	■				
Caesar salad dressing	1 Tbs		■				
Cake, angel food	1 oz	■					
Candy							
Crystallized ginger	2 tsp	■					
Hershey's Special Dark Chocolate	1.5 oz		■	■			
M & M's, milk chocolate	1.5 oz			■			
Peanut Butter Cup, Reese's	1.5 oz				■		
Raisinets	1.5 oz	■					
Snickers bar	1.5 oz		■				
Cannellini beans							
boiled	3.5 oz		■				
canned, unheated	3.5 oz		■				
raw	3.5 oz	■	■				
Canola oil	1 Tbs			■			
Cantaloupe							
grilled	3.5 oz	■	■				
raw	3.5 oz	■					

FOOD	Portion Size	Very Low 100 kU or less	Low 100–500 kU	Medium 501–1,000 kU	High 1,001–3,000 kU	Very High 3,001–5,000 kU	Highest 5,000–12,000 kU
Caramel syrup, sugar-free	1 Tbs	■					
Carnaroli rice	3.5 oz	■					
Carolina gold rice	3.5 oz	■					
Carrots							
baked	3.5 oz	■	■				
boiled	3.5 oz	■					
broiled	3.5 oz	■	■				
canned, unheated	3.5 oz	■					
grilled	3.5 oz	■	■				
raw	3.5 oz	■					
roasted	3.5 oz	■	■				
sautéed w/cooking spray	3.5 oz	■	■				
steamed	3.5 oz	■					
stir-fried w/cooking spray	3.5 oz	■	■				
Cashews							
raw	1 oz				■		
roasted	1 oz				■	■	
Casserole, tuna	3.5 oz		■				
Cauliflower							
baked	3.5 oz	■	■				
boiled	3.5 oz	■					
broiled	3.5 oz	■	■				
grilled	3.5 oz	■	■				
raw	3.5 oz	■					

FOOD	Portion Size	Very Low 100 kU or less	Low 100–500 kU	Medium 501–1,000 kU	High 1,001–3,000 kU	Very High 3,001–5,000 kU	Highest 5,000–12,000 kU
roasted	3.5 oz	■	■				
sautéed w/cooking spray	3.5 oz	■	■				
steamed	3.5 oz	■					
stir-fried w/cooking spray	3.5 oz	■	■				
Caviar spread, taramosalata	3.5 oz			■			
Celery							
boiled	3.5 oz	■					
broiled	3.5 oz	■	■				
grilled	3.5 oz	■	■				
raw	3.5 oz	■					
roasted	3.5 oz	■	■				
steamed	3.5 oz	■					
stir-fried w/cooking spray	3.5 oz	■	■				
Cereal, cooked							
Cream of Wheat	3/4 cup		■				
Cream of Wheat, w/honey	3/4 cup		■				
oatmeal	1 cup	■					
oatmeal, w/honey	1 cup	■					
Cereal, dry							
bran flakes	1 cup	■					
Cinnamon Toast Crunch	1 cup		■				
Corn Flakes	1 cup	■					

FOOD	Portion Size	Very Low 100 kU or less	Low 100–500 kU	Medium 501–1,000 kU	High 1,001–3,000 kU	Very High 3,001–5,000 kU	Highest 5,000–12,000 kU
Corn Pops	1 cup		■				
Honey Nut Cheerios	1 cup	■	■				
Fiber One	1 cup		■				
Froot Loops	1 cup	■					
Frosted Flakes	1 cup		■				
Frosted Mini Wheats	1 cup	■					
Granola, Organic Oats & Honey	2/3 cup		■				
Life	1 cup		■				
Puffed corn	1 cup	■					
Puffed wheat	1 cup	■					
Rice Krispies	1 cup			■			
Total, wheat and brown rice	1 cup	■					
Chanterelle mushrooms							
baked	3.5 oz	■	■				
boiled	3.5 oz	■					
broiled	3.5 oz	■	■				
grilled	3.5 oz	■	■				
raw	3.5 oz	■					
roasted	3.5 oz	■	■				
sautéed w/cooking spray	3.5 oz	■	■				
steamed	3.5 oz	■					
stir-fried w/cooking spray	3.5 oz	■	■				

FOOD	Portion Size	Very Low 100 kU or less	Low 100–500 kU	Medium 501–1,000 kU	High 1,001–3,000 kU	Very High 3,001–5,000 kU	Highest 5,000–12,000 kU
Chard, Swiss							
boiled	3.5 oz	■					
raw	3.5 oz	■					
sautéed w/cooking spray	3.5 oz	■	■				
steamed	3.5 oz	■					
stir-fried w/cooking spray	3.5 oz	■	■				
Cheddar cheese							
regular	1 oz				■		
white, 75% light	1 oz			■	■		
w/2% milk	1 oz			■			
Cheerios, Honey Nut	1 cup	■	■				

TIP

Enjoy cheese in moderate portions, and choose lower-fat products, as they tend to be lower in AGEs. If the cheese is to be melted, add it only during the last minute or two of cooking time. Browning cheese or placing it under the broiler will cause an explosion of AGEs.

FOOD	Portion Size	Very Low	Low	Medium	High	Very High	Highest
Cheese							
American	1 oz				■		
American, low-fat	1 oz			■	■		
brie	1 oz				■		
cheddar	1 oz				■		
cheddar, white, 75% light	1 oz			■	■		
cheddar, w/2% milk	1 oz			■			
cottage, 1% fat	1 oz		■				

FOOD	Portion Size	Very Low 100 kU or less	Low 100–500 kU	Medium 501–1,000 kU	High 1,001–3,000 kU	Very High 3,001–5,000 kU	Highest 5,000–12,000 kU
cream	1 oz				■		
feta, Greek, soft	1 oz				■		
mozzarella, fresh	1 oz		■	■			
mozzarella, part-skim	1 oz			■	■		
parmesan, grated	2 Tbs				■		
ricotta, part-skim	1 oz			■			
Swiss	1 oz				■		
Swiss, reduced-fat	1 oz			■	■		
Cheese Danish	2.5 oz			■			
Cheeseburger (fast food)	1 sandwich					■	
Cheeseburger, quarter-pound, double (fast food)	1 sandwich						■
Cheez Doodles, crunchy	1 oz			■			
Cherries							
cooked	3.5 oz	■					
raw	3.5 oz	■					
Chestnuts							
raw	1 oz			■			
roasted	1 oz				■		
Chex mix, traditional	1 oz		■				
Chicken, ground							
89% lean, raw	3 oz		■	■			
dark meat, w/skin, pan-fried	3 oz				■	■	

FOOD	Portion Size	Very Low 100 kU or less	Low 100–500 kU	Medium 501–1,000 kU	High 1,001–3,000 kU	Very High 3,001–5,000 kU	Highest 5,000–12,000 kU
dark meat, w/skin, raw	3 oz			■	■		
white meat, skinless, pan-fried	3 oz				■		
white meat, skinless, raw	3 oz			■			
Chicken bouillon	1 cup	■					

TIP

When you grill foods—which should be done only occasionally—an appliance such as the George Foreman Grill is a good choice. It cooks both sides at once, cutting cooking time in half, and also has a nonstick surface. Both of these properties help to control the formation of additional AGEs.

Chicken breast, skinless

FOOD	Portion Size	Very Low 100 kU or less	Low 100–500 kU	Medium 501–1,000 kU	High 1,001–3,000 kU	Very High 3,001–5,000 kU	Highest 5,000–12,000 kU
boiled	3 oz			■			
breaded, deep-fried	3 oz						■
breaded, pan-fried	3 oz						■
broiled	3 oz					■	■
grilled (nonstick grill)	3 oz					■	
marinated w/lemon, grilled (nonstick grill)	3 oz			■			
microwaved	3 oz				■		
oven-baked w/white wine in parchment	3 oz			■			
pan-fried	3 oz					■	
poached	3 oz			■			
raw	3 oz		■				

FOOD	Portion Size	Very Low 100 kU or less	Low 100–500 kU	Medium 501–1,000 kU	High 1,001–3,000 kU	Very High 3,001–5,000 kU	Highest 5,000–12,000 kU
roasted	3 oz					■	■
simmered	3 oz			■			
in slow-cooker	3 oz			■			
steamed in foil	3 oz			■			
Chicken breast, w/skin							
breaded, oven-fried	3 oz						■
broiled	3 oz						■
roasted	3 oz						■
Chicken breast strips							
stir-fried w/oil	3 oz					■	
stir-fried w/out oil	3 oz				■	■	
Chicken broth	1 cup	■					
Chicken burger, 89% lean							
pan-fried w/cooking spray	3 oz				■		
Chicken kebab w/skinless breast cubes							
pan-fried	3 oz					■	■
Chicken leg							
skinless, roasted	3 oz					■	
w/skin, roasted	3 oz						■
Chicken loaf, baked	3 oz				■	■	
Chicken noodle soup	1 cup	■					
Chicken nuggets, fried (fast food)	6 nuggets						■

FOOD	Portion Size	Very Low 100 kU or less	Low 100–500 kU	Medium 501–1,000 kU	High 1,001–3,000 kU	Very High 3,001–5,000 kU	Highest 5,000–12,000 kU
Chicken sandwich							
crispy (fast food)	1 sandwich						■
grilled (fast food)	1 sandwich						■
Chicken sausage, Italian, 96% lean							
pan-cooked	3 oz			■	■		
raw	3 oz			■			
Chicken thigh, w/skin, roasted	3 oz						■
Chicory (curly endive, frisee)	3.5 oz	■					
Chickpeas (garbanzo beans)							
boiled	3.5 oz		■				
canned, unheated	3.5 oz		■				
raw	3.5 oz	■	■				
Chinese black forbidden rice	3.5 oz	■					
Chips							
corn	1 oz		■				
plantain	1 oz		■				
potato	1 oz			■			
potato, baked	1 oz		■				
Chocolate candy, Special Dark (Hershey's)	1.5 oz		■	■			
Chocolate chip cookie	1 oz			■			

FOOD	Portion Size	Very Low 100 kU or less	Low 100–500 kU	Medium 501–1,000 kU	High 1,001–3,000 kU	Very High 3,001–5,000 kU	Highest 5,000–12,000 kU
Chocolate graham cracker	1 oz		■				
Cinnamon swirl sweet roll	2.5 oz			■			
Cinnamon Toast Crunch cereal	1 cup		■				
Clementine	3.5 oz	■					
Coca Cola							
classic	8 oz	■					
diet	8 oz	■					
Cocoa (Swiss Miss)							
regular	1 cup			■			
sugar-free (Swiss Miss)	1 cup		■	■			
Coconut cream	1 Tbs	■	■				
Coconut flakes, sweetened	1 oz		■				
Coconut milk	1/3 cup		■				
Coffee							
instant	1 cup	■					
instant, decaf	1 cup	■					
regular	1 cup	■					
Spanish	1 cup	■					
w/milk	1 cup	■					
w/sugar	1 cup	■					
Coke. ***See*** **Coca Cola.**							
Collard greens							
baked	3.5 oz	■	■				

FOOD	Portion Size	Very Low 100 kU or less	Low 100–500 kU	Medium 501–1,000 kU	High 1,001–3,000 kU	Very High 3,001–5,000 kU	Highest 5,000–12,000 kU
boiled	3.5 oz	■					
raw	3.5 oz	■					
sautéed w/cooking spray	3.5 oz	■	■				
steamed	3.5 oz	■					
stir-fried w/cooking spray	3.5 oz	■	■				
Combos, nacho cheese pretzel	1 oz			■			

TIP

When you want to indulge, choose a relatively low-AGE dessert—a dairy treat such as ice cream or pudding, or a fruit dessert such as sorbet or grilled fruit. When sweeteners are added to other ingredients and heated—when you bake cakes or cookies, for instance—they can react with proteins and fats to form AGEs.

FOOD	Portion Size	Very Low 100 kU or less	Low 100–500 kU	Medium 501–1,000 kU	High 1,001–3,000 kU	Very High 3,001–5,000 kU	Highest 5,000–12,000 kU
Cookie							
biscotti, vanilla almond	1 oz			■			
chocolate chip	1 oz			■			
fortune	1 oz	■					
meringue	1 oz		■				
oatmeal raisin	1 oz		■				
Oreo	1 oz			■			
vanilla wafer	1 oz		■				
Corn							
baked	3.5 oz	■	■				
boiled	3.5 oz	■					
broiled	3.5 oz	■	■				

FOOD	Portion Size	Very Low 100 kU or less	Low 100–500 kU	Medium 501–1,000 kU	High 1,001–3,000 kU	Very High 3,001–5,000 kU	Highest 5,000–12,000 kU
canned, unheated	3.5 oz	■					
grilled	3.5 oz	■	■				
microwaved	3.5 oz	■					
raw	3.5 oz	■					
roasted	3.5 oz	■	■				
sautéed w/cooking spray	3.5 oz	■	■				
steamed	3.5 oz	■					
stir-fried w/cooking spray	3.5 oz	■	■				
Corn chips	1 oz		■				
Corn Flakes cereal							
plain	1 cup	■					
frosted	1 cup		■				
Corn oil	1 Tbs				■		
Corn Pops cereal	1 cup		■				
Corn syrup, dark	1 Tbs	■					
Corned beef, low-fat	3 oz			■			
Corned beef hash, canned							
microwaved	3.5 oz				■		
pan-heated	3.5 oz				■		
unheated	3.5 oz			■	■		
Cos lettuce (romaine)	3.5 oz	■					
Cottage cheese, 1% fat	1 oz		■				
Cottonseed oil	1 Tbs			■	■		

FOOD	Portion Size	Very Low 100 kU or less	Low 100–500 kU	Medium 501–1,000 kU	High 1,001–3,000 kU	Very High 3,001–5,000 kU	Highest 5,000–12,000 kU
Courgette (zucchini)							
baked	3.5 oz	■	■				
boiled	3.5 oz	■					
broiled	3.5 oz	■	■				
grilled	3.5 oz	■	■				
raw	3.5 oz	■					
roasted	3.5 oz	■	■				
sautéed w/cooking spray	3.5 oz	■	■				
steamed	3.5 oz	■					
stir-fried w/cooking spray	3.5 oz	■	■				
Couscous	3.5 oz		■				
Couscous and lentil soup	1 cup	■					
Crabmeat							
boiled	3 oz		■				
breaded, fried	3 oz					■	
Cracker							
chocolate graham	1 oz		■				
goldfish, cheddar	1 oz			■			
honey graham	1 oz		■				
melba toast	1 oz		■				
oyster	1 oz			■			
rice cake, corn flavored	1 oz	■					
rice crunch	1 oz		■				
saltine	1 oz		■				

FOOD	Portion Size	Very Low 100 kU or less	Low 100–500 kU	Medium 501–1,000 kU	High 1,001–3,000 kU	Very High 3,001–5,000 kU	Highest 5,000–12,000 kU
sandwich (club crackers w/cheddar)	1 oz			■			
toasted wheat	1 oz		■				
wheat	1 oz		■				

TIP

Substitute wedges of whole grain pita bread or rounds of whole grain bagels for crackers, as bread contains less AGEs than crackers. Even better, use Belgian endive leaves and other fresh vegetables to scoop up dips and spreads.

FOOD	Portion Size	Very Low 100 kU or less	Low 100–500 kU	Medium 501–1,000 kU	High 1,001–3,000 kU	Very High 3,001–5,000 kU	Highest 5,000–12,000 kU
Cranberries							
cooked	3.5 oz	■					
raw	3.5 oz	■					
Cranberry juice	8 oz	■					
Cream, coconut	1 Tbs	■	■				
Cream, heavy, ultra-pasteurized	1 Tbs		■				
Cream cheese	1 oz				■		
Cream of celery soup, low-fat	1 cup		■				
Cream of Wheat, instant							
regular	3/4 cup		■				
w/honey	3/4 cup		■				
Crenshaw melon							
grilled	3.5 oz	■	■				
raw	3.5 oz	■					

FOOD	Portion Size	Very Low 100 kU or less	Low 100–500 kU	Medium 501–1,000 kU	High 1,001–3,000 kU	Very High 3,001–5,000 kU	Highest 5,000–12,000 kU
Cress (watercress)	3.5 oz	■					
Crimini mushrooms (baby bella)							
baked	3.5 oz	■	■				
boiled	3.5 oz	■					
broiled	3.5 oz	■	■				
grilled	3.5 oz	■	■				
raw	3.5 oz	■					
roasted	3.5 oz	■	■				
sautéed w/cooking spray	3.5 oz	■	■				
steamed	3.5 oz	■					
stir-fried w/cooking spray	3.5 oz	■	■				
Crispy chicken sandwich (fast food)	1 sandwich						■
Croissant, classic butter	2 oz			■			
Cucumber							
baked	3.5 oz	■	■				
grilled	3.5 oz	■	■				
raw	3.5 oz	■					
roasted	3.5 oz	■	■				
stir-fried w/cooking spray	3.5 oz	■	■				
Curly endive (chicory, frisee)	3.5 oz	■					
Currants							
cooked	3.5 oz	■					

FOOD	Portion Size	Very Low 100 kU or less	Low 100–500 kU	Medium 501–1,000 kU	High 1,001–3,000 kU	Very High 3,001–5,000 kU	Highest 5,000–12,000 kU
raw	3.5 oz	■					
Dandelion greens							
boiled	3.5 oz	■					
raw	3.5 oz	■					
sautéed w/cooking spray	3.5 oz	■	■				
steamed	3.5 oz	■					
stir-fried w/cooking spray	3.5 oz	■	■				
Danish, cheese	2.5 oz			■			
Dark Chocolate, Special (Hershey's)	1.5 oz		■	■			
Dates, chopped	1 oz	■					
Donut							
chocolate iced, cream-filled	2.5 oz			■	■		
devil's food cake, glazed	2.5 oz			■	■		
Double quarter-pound cheeseburger (fast food)	1 sandwich						■
Dutch Apple Crumb Pie (Mrs. Smith's)	1/8 pie			■			
Edamame							
boiled	3.5 oz	■					
steamed	3.5 oz	■					
Egg, fried	1 large				■		
Egg, poached	1 large	■					

FOOD	Portion Size	Very Low 100 kU or less	Low 100–500 kU	Medium 501–1,000 kU	High 1,001–3,000 kU	Very High 3,001–5,000 kU	Highest 5,000–12,000 kU
Egg, scrambled							
w/butter	1 large		■				
w/cooking spray	1 large	■					
w/corn oil	1 large	■					
w/margarine	1 large	■					
w/olive oil	1 large	■					

TIP

Enjoy eggs as a high-nutrient, low-AGE source of protein. To keep AGE formation at the lowest possible level, poach your eggs or scramble them over gentle heat. Avoid frying, as this raises AGE levels.

FOOD	Portion Size	Very Low 100 kU or less	Low 100–500 kU	Medium 501–1,000 kU	High 1,001–3,000 kU	Very High 3,001–5,000 kU	Highest 5,000–12,000 kU
Egg omelet							
w/butter	1 large		■				
w/cooking spray	1 large	■					
w/corn oil	1 large	■					
w/margarine	1 large	■					
w/olive oil	1 large	■					
Egg substitute omelet, w/cooking spray	1/4 cup	■					
Egg white, hard boiled	1 large	■					
Egg yolk, hard boiled	1 large		■				
Eggplant (aubergine)							
baked	3.5 oz	■	■				
broiled	3.5 oz	■	■				
grilled	3.5 oz	■	■				

FOOD	Portion Size	Very Low 100 kU or less	Low 100–500 kU	Medium 501–1,000 kU	High 1,001–3,000 kU	Very High 3,001–5,000 kU	Highest 5,000–12,000 kU
raw	3.5 oz	■					
roasted	3.5 oz	■	■				
sautéed w/cooking spray	3.5 oz	■	■				
steamed	3.5 oz	■					
stewed	3.5 oz	■					
stir-fried w/cooking spray	3.5 oz	■	■				
Elderberries							
cooked	3.5 oz	■					
raw	3.5 oz	■					
Emmer	3.5 oz	■					
Endive (Belgian endive, witloof)	3.5 oz	■					
Enfamil infant formula	2 Tbs		■				
Enoki mushrooms							
baked	3.5 oz	■	■				
boiled	3.5 oz	■					
broiled	3.5 oz	■	■				
grilled	3.5 oz	■	■				
raw	3.5 oz	■					
roasted	3.5 oz	■	■				
sautéed w/cooking spray	3.5 oz	■	■				
steamed	3.5 oz	■					
stir-fried w/cooking spray	3.5 oz	■	■				
Ensure Plus nutrition drink	8 oz	■					

FOOD	Portion Size	Very Low 100 kU or less	Low 100–500 kU	Medium 501–1,000 kU	High 1,001–3,000 kU	Very High 3,001–5,000 kU	Highest 5,000–12,000 kU
Escarole							
boiled	3.5 oz	■					
raw	3.5 oz	■					
sautéed w/cooking spray	3.5 oz	■	■				
steamed							
stir-fried w/cooking spray	3.5 oz	■	■				
Farro	3.5 oz	■					
Fava beans							
boiled	3.5 oz		■				
raw	3.5 oz	■	■				
Feta cheese, soft, Greek	1 oz				■		
Fiber One cereal	1 cup		■				
Fig, fresh							
grilled	3.5 oz	■	■				
raw	3.5 oz	■					
Fish/Seafood. ***See*** **individual varieties.**							
Fish loaf (gefilte), boiled	3 oz			■			
Fish sandwich, fried (fast food)	1 sandwich						■
Flounder							
oven-baked in parchment w/tomatoes	3 oz		■	■			
pan-cooked (nonstick), w/cooking spray	3 oz			■			
raw	3 oz		■				

FOOD	Portion Size	Very Low 100 kU or less	Low 100–500 kU	Medium 501–1,000 kU	High 1,001–3,000 kU	Very High 3,001–5,000 kU	Highest 5,000–12,000 kU
Forbidden black rice, Chinese	3.5 oz	■					
Fortune cookie	1 oz	■					

TIP

To reduce AGE formation during cooking, marinate meat, poultry, and seafood in low-sugar, low-oil marinades made with acidic ingredients such as lemon juice, lime juice, tomato juice, vinegar, and wine. To increase the food's absorption of the marinade and speed cooking time, cut the food into small pieces for kebabs or "butterfly" it to create a thinner cut.

FOOD	Portion Size	Very Low	Low	Medium	High	Very High	Highest
Frankfurter, beef							
boiled	3 oz					■	■
broiled	3 oz						■
French fries, cooked in corn oil	3.5 oz			■			
French fries (fast food)							
small	2.5 oz			■	■		
medium	4 oz				■		
large	6 oz				■	■	
French salad dressing							
lite	1 Tbs	■					
regular	1 Tbs	■	■				
French toast, frozen (Aunt Jemima)							
in toaster oven	1 slice		■				
microwaved	1 slice		■				
not heated	1 slice	■	■				

FOOD	Portion Size	Very Low 100 kU or less	Low 100–500 kU	Medium 501–1,000 kU	High 1,001–3,000 kU	Very High 3,001–5,000 kU	Highest 5,000–12,000 kU
French toast, whole grain, low-fat	1 slice	■	■				
Frisee (chicory, curly endive)	3.5 oz	■					
Froot Loops cereal	1 cup	■					
Frosted Flakes cereal	1 cup		■				
Frosted Mini Wheats cereal	1 cup	■					

TIP

Whenever possible, satisfy your sweet tooth with whole fresh fruit. It's low in AGEs and high in vitamins, minerals, and fiber.

FOOD	Portion Size	Very Low 100 kU or less	Low 100–500 kU	Medium 501–1,000 kU	High 1,001–3,000 kU	Very High 3,001–5,000 kU	Highest 5,000–12,000 kU
Fruit. ***See*** **individual varieties.**							
Fruit pop, frozen	2 oz	■					
Fruit roll-up	1 oz		■				
Garbanzo beans (chickpeas)							
boiled	3.5 oz		■				
canned, unheated	3.5 oz		■				
raw	3.5 oz	■	■				
Garlic							
raw	1 oz	■					
roasted	1 oz	■	■				
sautéed w/cooking spray	1 oz	■	■				
stir-fried w/cooking spray	1 oz	■	■				
Gefilte fish (fish loaf), boiled	3 oz			■			

FOOD	Portion Size	Very Low 100 kU or less	Low 100–500 kU	Medium 501–1,000 kU	High 1,001–3,000 kU	Very High 3,001–5,000 kU	Highest 5,000–12,000 kU
Gelatin, fruit-flavored							
regular	1/2 cup	■					
sugar-free	1/2 cup	■					
Gin	1.5 oz	■					
Ginger							
crystallized	2 tsp	■					
raw, grated	2 tsp	■					
Glazed donut, devil's food	2.5 oz			■	■		
Glucerna nutrition drink	8 oz		■				
Gnocchi, potato, w/parmesan cheese	3.5 oz			■			
Goji berries	3.5 oz	■					
Goldfish cracker, cheddar	1 oz			■			
Graham cracker							
chocolate	1 oz		■				
honey	1 oz		■				
Grains. *See* individual varieties.							
Granola, Organic Oats & Honey cereal (Cascadian Farms)	2/3 cup		■				
Granola bar							
Chocolate Chunk (Quaker)	1 bar		■				
Peanut Butter/Chocolate Chip (Quaker)	1 bar			■			

FOOD	Portion Size	Very Low 100 kU or less	Low 100–500 kU	Medium 501–1,000 kU	High 1,001–3,000 kU	Very High 3,001–5,000 kU	Highest 5,000–12,000 kU
Granola cereal, Organic Oats & Honey (Cascadian Farms)	$^{2}/_{3}$ cup		■				
Granulated sugar	1 tsp	■					
Grapefruit	3.5 oz	■					
Grapes							
cooked	3.5 oz	■					
raw	3.5 oz	■					
Great Northern beans							
boiled	3.5 oz		■				
canned, unheated	3.5 oz		■				
raw	3.5 oz	■	■				
Green beans							
baked	3.5 oz	■	■				
boiled	3.5 oz	■					
canned, unheated	3.5 oz	■					
raw	3.5 oz	■					
sautéed w/cooking spray	3.5 oz	■	■				
steamed	3.5 oz	■					

TIP

Boiled and steamed whole grains such as brown rice, barley, farro, and quinoa are low in AGEs and high in fiber and nutrients, making them an important part of a healthy diet. To reduce carb and calorie counts, toss plenty of vegetables into your grain-based salads, side dishes, and casseroles.

FOOD	Portion Size	Very Low 100 kU or less	Low 100–500 kU	Medium 501–1,000 kU	High 1,001–3,000 kU	Very High 3,001–5,000 kU	Highest 5,000–12,000 kU
stir-fried w/cooking spray	3.5 oz	■	■				
Green onion (scallion)							
boiled	3.5 oz	■					
broiled	3.5 oz	■	■				
grilled	3.5 oz	■	■				
raw	3.5 oz	■					
roasted	3.5 oz	■	■				
sautéed w/cooking spray	3.5 oz	■	■				
steamed	3.5 oz	■					
stir-fried w/cooking spray	3.5 oz	■	■				
Greens, collard							
baked	3.5 oz	■	■				
boiled	3.5 oz	■					
raw	3.5 oz	■					
sautéed w/cooking spray	3.5 oz	■	■				
steamed	3.5 oz	■					
stir-fried w/cooking spray	3.5 oz	■	■				
Greens, dandelion							
boiled	3.5 oz	■					
raw	3.5 oz	■					
sautéed w/cooking spray	3.5 oz	■	■				
steamed	3.5 oz	■					
stir-fried w/cooking spray	3.5 oz	■	■				

FOOD	Portion Size	Very Low 100 kU or less	Low 100–500 kU	Medium 501–1,000 kU	High 1,001–3,000 kU	Very High 3,001–5,000 kU	Highest 5,000–12,000 kU
Greens, mustard							
boiled	3.5 oz	■					
raw	3.5 oz	■					
sautéed w/cooking spray	3.5 oz	■	■				
steamed	3.5 oz	■					
stir-fried w/cooking spray	3.5 oz	■	■				
Grilled chicken sandwich (fast food)	1 sandwich						■
Grits	3.5 oz	■					

TIP

A good way to fit ground beef into a low-AGE diet is to mix in chopped mushrooms. Meaty tasting and low in AGEs, mushrooms boost nutritional value and make meat portions go further. Replace up to a third of the meat in meatballs, burgers, and meatloaf, and up to half of the meat in tacos.

FOOD	Portion Size	Very Low	Low	Medium	High	Very High	Highest
Ground beef							
80% lean, pan-browned	3 oz					■	
91% lean, grass-fed, pan-browned	3 oz			■			
91% lean, grass-fed, raw	3 oz		■				
93% lean, pan-browned	3 oz			■	■		
93% lean, raw	3 oz			■			
Grouper							
grilled (nonstick grill), w/cooking spray	3 oz			■			
raw	3 oz		■				

FOOD	Portion Size	Very Low 100 kU or less	Low 100–500 kU	Medium 501–1,000 kU	High 1,001–3,000 kU	Very High 3,001–5,000 kU	Highest 5,000–12,000 kU
Ham, deli							
smoked	3 oz				■		
Virginia	3 oz			■			
Hamburger patty, beef (fast food)	3 oz					■	
Hamburger patty, beef, 93% lean							
grilled (nonstick grill)	3 oz				■		
pan-cooked	3 oz				■		
Hash, corned beef, canned							
microwaved	3.5 oz				■		
pan-heated	3.5 oz				■		
unheated	3.5 oz			■	■		
Hash brown potatoes (fast food)	2 oz	■	■				
Hershey's Special Dark Chocolate	1.5 oz		■	■			
Honey	1 Tbs	■					
Honey graham cracker	1 oz		■				
Honey Nut Cheerios	1 cup	■	■				
Honeydew melon							
grilled	3.5 oz	■	■				
raw	3.5 oz	■					
Hot dog, beef							
boiled	3 oz					■	■
broiled	3 oz						■

FOOD	Portion Size	Very Low 100 kU or less	Low 100–500 kU	Medium 501–1,000 kU	High 1,001–3,000 kU	Very High 3,001–5,000 kU	Highest 5,000–12,000 kU
Hot Pocket, Bacon, Egg & Cheese							
microwaved	1 pocket			■	■		
not heated	1 pocket			■			
oven-baked	1 pocket				■		
Hotcakes (McDonald's)	3 hot-cakes		■				
Huckleberries							
cooked	3.5 oz	■					
raw	3.5 oz	■					
Hummus	3.5 oz			■			
Ice cream, vanilla	1 cup	■					
Ice cream cone, sugar (cone only)	1 oz	■					
Ice cream cone, waffle (cone only)	1 oz	■					
Iceberg lettuce	3.5 oz	■					
Italian salad dressing							
lite	1 Tbs	■					
regular	1 Tbs	■	■				
Japonica rice, black	3.5 oz	■					
Jasmine rice	3.5 oz	■					
Jerky, meatless	3 oz				■		
Jicama							
baked	3.5 oz	■	■				

FOOD	Portion Size	Very Low 100 kU or less	Low 100–500 kU	Medium 501–1,000 kU	High 1,001–3,000 kU	Very High 3,001–5,000 kU	Highest 5,000–12,000 kU
boiled	3.5 oz	■					
raw	3.5 oz	■					
roasted	3.5 oz	■	■				
sautéed w/cooking spray	3.5 oz	■	■				
steamed	3.5 oz	■					
stir-fried w/cooking spray	3.5 oz	■	■				
Juice							
apple	8 oz	■					
cranberry	8 oz	■					
orange	8 oz	■					
orange, w/calcium	8 oz	■					
vegetable	8 oz	■					
Kale							
baked	3.5 oz	■	■				
boiled	3.5 oz	■					
raw	3.5 oz	■					
roasted	3.5 oz	■	■				
sautéed w/cooking spray	3.5 oz	■	■				
steamed	3.5 oz	■					
stir-fried w/cooking spray	3.5 oz	■	■				
Kamut	3.5 oz	■					
Kebab, chicken, w/skinless breast cubes, pan-fried	3 oz				■	■	

FOOD	Portion Size	Very Low 100 kU or less	Low 100–500 kU	Medium 501–1,000 kU	High 1,001–3,000 kU	Very High 3,001–5,000 kU	Highest 5,000–12,000 kU
Ketchup	1 Tbs	■					
Kidney beans, red							
boiled	3.5 oz		■				
canned, unheated	3.5 oz		■				
raw	3.5 oz	■	■				

TIP

Skip high-sugar condiments like ketchup and sweet barbecue sauce. Although they are low in AGEs, because of their high sugar content, these products can boost AGE levels if used in excess and on a frequent basis.

FOOD	Portion Size	Very Low 100 kU or less	Low 100–500 kU	Medium 501–1,000 kU	High 1,001–3,000 kU	Very High 3,001–5,000 kU	Highest 5,000–12,000 kU
Kiwifruit	3.5 oz	■					
Kumquat							
grilled	3.5 oz	■	■				
raw	3.5 oz	■					
roasted	3.5 oz	■	■				
Lamb, from leg							
boiled	3 oz			■	■		
broiled	3 oz				■		
microwaved	3 oz			■	■		
raw	3 oz			■			
Leeks							
baked	3.5 oz	■	■				
boiled	3.5 oz	■					
broiled	3.5 oz	■	■				

FOOD	Portion Size	Very Low 100 kU or less	Low 100–500 kU	Medium 501–1,000 kU	High 1,001–3,000 kU	Very High 3,001–5,000 kU	Highest 5,000–12,000 kU
grilled	3.5 oz	■	■				
raw	3.5 oz	■					
roasted	3.5 oz	■	■				
sautéed w/cooking spray	3.5 oz	■	■				
steamed	3.5 oz	■					
stir-fried w/cooking spray	3.5 oz	■	■				
Leeks, wild (ramps)							
baked	3.5 oz	■	■				
boiled	3.5 oz	■					
broiled	3.5 oz	■	■				
grilled	3.5 oz	■	■				
raw	3.5 oz	■					
roasted	3.5 oz	■	■				
sautéed w/cooking spray	3.5 oz	■	■				
steamed	3.5 oz	■					
stir-fried w/cooking spray	3.5 oz	■	■				

TIP

To trim AGEs from your diet, enjoy legumes—beans, peas, and lentils—as often as possible. In addition to being low in AGEs, legumes are inexpensive, super-nutritious, and highly versatile.

Legumes/Beans. *See* individual varieties.

FOOD	Portion Size	Very Low 100 kU or less	Low 100–500 kU	Medium 501–1,000 kU	High 1,001–3,000 kU	Very High 3,001–5,000 kU	Highest 5,000–12,000 kU
Lemon	3.5 oz	■					
Lentil soup, vegetarian	1 cup		■				

FOOD	Portion Size	Very Low 100 kU or less	Low 100–500 kU	Medium 501–1,000 kU	High 1,001–3,000 kU	Very High 3,001–5,000 kU	Highest 5,000–12,000 kU
Lentils							
boiled	3.5 oz		■				
canned, unheated	3.5 oz		■				
raw	3.5 oz	■	■				
Lettuce, all varieties	3.5 oz	■					
Life cereal	1 cup		■				
Lima beans							
boiled	3.5 oz		■				
canned, unheated	3.5 oz		■				
raw	3.5 oz	■	■				
Lime	3.5 oz	■					
Liverwurst	3 oz			■			
Loganberries							
cooked	3.5 oz	■					
raw	3.5 oz	■					
M & M's, milk chocolate	1.5 oz			■			
Macaroni and cheese, baked	3.5 oz				■	■	
Mache salad greens	3.5 oz	■					
Malta malt beverage	8 oz	■					
Mango							
baked	3.5 oz	■	■				
grilled	3.5 oz	■	■				
raw	3.5 oz	■					

FOOD	Portion Size	Very Low 100 kU or less	Low 100–500 kU	Medium 501–1,000 kU	High 1,001–3,000 kU	Very High 3,001–5,000 kU	Highest 5,000–12,000 kU
Margarine	1 Tbs			■	■		
Mayonnaise							
fat-free	1 Tbs	■					
low-fat	1 Tbs		■				
regular	1 Tbs			■			
Meat. *See* individual varieties.							
Meatball, beef							
simmered in broth	3 oz					■	
93% lean, simmered in tomato sauce	3 oz				■		
Meatloaf, beef							
oven-baked	3 oz				■		
93% lean, oven-baked	3 oz			■			
Melba toast	1 oz		■				
Meringue cookie	1 oz		■				

TIP

Nonfat, reduced-fat, and whole milk are all low in AGEs. To trim calories and saturated fat, choose the lower-fat varieties most often. Save whole milk for coffee or recipes in which you want to add richness. Avoid cream, which contains many more AGEs than milk.

FOOD	Portion Size	Very Low 100 kU or less	Low 100–500 kU	Medium 501–1,000 kU	High 1,001–3,000 kU	Very High 3,001–5,000 kU	Highest 5,000–12,000 kU
Milk							
fat-free	1 cup	■					
fat-free w/vitamins A and D	1 cup	■					

FOOD	Portion Size	Very Low 100 kU or less	Low 100–500 kU	Medium 501–1,000 kU	High 1,001–3,000 kU	Very High 3,001–5,000 kU	Highest 5,000–12,000 kU
reduced fat	1 cup	■					
soy	1 cup	■					
whole	1 cup	■					
Milk, breast							
fresh	1 oz	■					
frozen	1 oz	■					
Milk, coconut	1/3 cup		■				
Mizuna salad greens	3.5 oz	■					
Morel mushrooms							
baked	3.5 oz	■	■				
boiled	3.5 oz	■					
broiled	3.5 oz	■	■				
grilled	3.5 oz	■	■				
raw	3.5 oz	■					
roasted	3.5 oz	■	■				
sautéed w/cooking spray	3.5 oz	■	■				
steamed	3.5 oz	■					
stir-fried w/cooking spray	3.5 oz	■	■				
Mozzarella cheese							
fresh	1 oz		■	■			
part-skim	1 oz			■	■		
Muffin, bran	2.5 oz		■				
Mulberries							
cooked	3.5 oz	■					

FOOD	Portion Size	Very Low 100 kU or less	Low 100–500 kU	Medium 501–1,000 kU	High 1,001–3,000 kU	Very High 3,001–5,000 kU	Highest 5,000–12,000 kU
raw	3.5 oz	■					
Mushrooms, all varieties							
baked	3.5 oz	■	■				
boiled	3.5 oz	■					
broiled	3.5 oz	■	■				
grilled	3.5 oz	■	■				
raw	3.5 oz	■					
roasted	3.5 oz	■	■				
sautéed w/cooking spray	3.5 oz	■	■				
steamed	3.5 oz	■					
stir-fried w/cooking spray	3.5 oz	■	■				
Mustard	1 Tbs	■					
Mustard greens							
boiled	3.5 oz	■					
raw	3.5 oz	■					
sautéed w/cooking spray	3.5 oz	■	■				
steamed	3.5 oz	■					
stir-fried w/cooking spray	3.5 oz	■	■				
Navy beans							
boiled	3.5 oz		■				
canned, unheated	3.5 oz		■				
raw	3.5 oz	■	■				
Nectarine							
baked	3.5 oz	■	■				

FOOD	Portion Size	Very Low 100 kU or less	Low 100–500 kU	Medium 501–1,000 kU	High 1,001–3,000 kU	Very High 3,001–5,000 kU	Highest 5,000–12,000 kU
grilled	3.5 oz	■	■				
poached	3.5 oz	■					
raw	3.5 oz	■					
Nuggets, chicken, fried (fast food)	6 nuggets						■
Nutrigrain bar, Apple Cinnamon	1 bar			■			
Nuts. *See* individual varieties.							
Oatmeal, instant							
plain	1 cup	■					
w/honey	1 cup	■					
Oatmeal raisin cookie	1 oz		■				
Oats	3.5 oz	■					

TIP

Keep in mind that when it comes to fats and oils, the AGE content can vary greatly. This variation depends on such factors as the product's age and whether it has been exposed to air, light, and/or heat—all of which increase oxidation and AGEs.

FOOD	Portion Size	Very Low	Low	Medium	High	Very High	Highest
Oil							
canola	1 Tbs			■			
corn	1 Tbs				■		
cottonseed	1 Tbs			■	■		
olive	1 Tbs		■				
peanut	1 Tbs				■		
safflower	1 Tbs		■	■			

FOOD	Portion Size	Very Low 100 kU or less	Low 100–500 kU	Medium 501–1,000 kU	High 1,001–3,000 kU	Very High 3,001–5,000 kU	Highest 5,000–12,000 kU
sesame	1 Tbs		■				
sesame, toasted	1 Tbs					■	
sunflower	1 Tbs			■			
Okra							
boiled	3.5 oz	■					
broiled	3.5 oz	■	■				
grilled	3.5 oz	■	■				
roasted	3.5 oz	■	■				
steamed	3.5 oz	■					
Olive oil	1 Tbs		■				
Olives, ripe	1 oz			■			
Omelet, egg							
w/butter	1 large		■				
w/cooking spray	1 large	■					
w/corn oil	1 large	■					
w/margarine	1 large	■					
w/olive oil	1 large	■					
Omelet, egg substitute, w/cooking spray	$^{1}/_{4}$ cup	■					
Onion							
baked	3.5 oz	■	■				
boiled	3.5 oz	■					
broiled	3.5 oz	■	■				
grilled	3.5 oz	■	■				

FOOD	Portion Size	Very Low 100 kU or less	Low 100–500 kU	Medium 501–1,000 kU	High 1,001–3,000 kU	Very High 3,001–5,000 kU	Highest 5,000–12,000 kU
raw	3.5 oz	■					
roasted	3.5 oz	■	■				
sautéed w/cooking spray	3.5 oz	■	■				
steamed	3.5 oz	■					
stir-fried w/cooking spray	3.5 oz	■	■				
Onion, green (scallion)							
baked	3.5 oz	■	■				
boiled	3.5 oz	■					
broiled	3.5 oz	■	■				
grilled	3.5 oz	■	■				
raw	3.5 oz	■					
roasted	3.5 oz	■	■				
sautéed w/cooking spray	3.5 oz	■	■				
steamed	3.5 oz	■					
stir-fried w/cooking spray	3.5 oz	■	■				
Orange	3.5 oz	■					
Orange juice							
regular	8 oz	■					
w/calcium	8 oz	■					
Oreo cookie	1 oz			■			
Oyster cracker	1 oz			■			
Oyster mushrooms							
baked	3.5 oz	■	■				
boiled	3.5 oz	■					

FOOD	Portion Size	Very Low 100 kU or less	Low 100–500 kU	Medium 501–1,000 kU	High 1,001–3,000 kU	Very High 3,001–5,000 kU	Highest 5,000–12,000 kU
broiled	3.5 oz	■	■				
grilled	3.5 oz	■	■				
raw	3.5 oz	■					
roasted	3.5 oz	■	■				
sautéed w/cooking spray	3.5 oz	■	■				
steamed	3.5 oz	■					
stir-fried w/cooking spray	3.5 oz	■	■				
Pancake							
from mix	1 oz		■				
frozen, toasted	1 oz			■			
Pancake syrup							
lite	1 Tbs	■					
regular	1 Tbs	■					
Papaya							
baked	3.5 oz	■	■				
grilled	3.5 oz	■	■				
raw	3.5 oz	■					
Parmesan cheese, grated	2 Tbs				■		
Parsnip							
baked	3.5 oz	■	■				
boiled	3.5 oz	■					
raw	3.5 oz	■					
roasted	3.5 oz	■	■				
sautéed w/cooking spray	3.5 oz	■	■				

FOOD	Portion Size	Very Low 100 kU or less	Low 100–500 kU	Medium 501–1,000 kU	High 1,001–3,000 kU	Very High 3,001–5,000 kU	Highest 5,000–12,000 kU
steamed	3.5 oz	■					
stir-fried w/cooking spray	3.5 oz	■	■				
Passion fruit							
cooked	3.5 oz	■					
raw	3.5 oz	■					
Pasta							
cooked al dente (7–8 minutes)	3.5 oz	■	■				
cooked well (11–12 minutes)	3.5 oz		■				
Pasta primavera	3.5 oz			■			
Pasta salad							
Italian	3.5 oz			■			
tuna	3.5 oz		■				
Peach							
baked	3.5 oz	■	■				
grilled	3.5 oz	■	■				
poached	3.5 oz	■					
raw	3.5 oz	■					
Peanut butter, smooth	2 Tbs				■		
Peanut Butter Cup (Reese's)	1.5 oz				■		
Peanut oil	1 Tbs				■		
Peanuts							
cocktail	1 oz				■		

FOOD	Portion Size	Very Low 100 kU or less	Low 100–500 kU	Medium 501–1,000 kU	High 1,001–3,000 kU	Very High 3,001–5,000 kU	Highest 5,000–12,000 kU
dry roasted, unsalted	1 oz				■		
roasted in shell, salted	1 oz			■	■		
Pear							
baked	3.5 oz	■	■				
grilled	3.5 oz	■	■				
poached	3.5 oz	■					
raw	3.5 oz	■					

TIP

To minimize AGE formation when sautéing vegetables, use a nonstick pan and either cooking spray or a small amount of olive oil—no more than a teaspoon per serving. This will help keep AGE counts in the "Low" or even the "Very Low" range. Using larger amounts of oil can drive the AGE count up to unhealthy levels.

FOOD	Portion Size	Very Low	Low	Medium	High	Very High	Highest
Peas, black-eyed							
boiled	3.5 oz		■				
canned, unheated	3.5 oz		■				
raw	3.5 oz	■	■				
Peas, fresh							
boiled	3.5 oz	■					
canned, unheated	3.5 oz	■					
raw	3.5 oz	■					
sautéed w/cooking spray	3.5 oz	■	■				
steamed	3.5 oz	■					
stir-fried w/cooking spray	3.5 oz	■	■				

FOOD	Portion Size	Very Low 100 kU or less	Low 100–500 kU	Medium 501–1,000 kU	High 1,001–3,000 kU	Very High 3,001–5,000 kU	Highest 5,000–12,000 kU
Peas, snap							
boiled	3.5 oz	■					
raw	3.5 oz	■					
sautéed w/cooking spray	3.5 oz	■	■				
steamed	3.5 oz	■					
stir-fried w/cooking spray	3.5 oz	■	■				
Peas, snow							
boiled	3.5 oz	■					
raw	3.5 oz	■					
sautéed w/cooking spray	3.5 oz	■	■				
steamed	3.5 oz	■					
stir-fried w/cooking spray	3.5 oz	■	■				
Peas, split							
boiled	3.5 oz		■				
canned, unheated	3.5 oz		■				
raw	3.5 oz	■	■				
Pectin	1 Tbs	■					
Pepper, bell							
grilled	3.5 oz	■	■				
raw	3.5 oz	■					
roasted	3.5 oz	■	■				
sautéed w/cooking spray	3.5 oz	■	■				
steamed	3.5 oz	■					
stir-fried w/cooking spray	3.5 oz	■	■				

FOOD	Portion Size	Very Low 100 kU or less	Low 100–500 kU	Medium 501–1,000 kU	High 1,001–3,000 kU	Very High 3,001–5,000 kU	Highest 5,000–12,000 kU
Pepsi							
diet	8 oz	■					
diet, caffeine-free	8 oz	■					
regular	8 oz	■					
Persimmon							
cooked	3.5 oz	■					
raw	3.5 oz	■					
Pesto, with basil	1 Tbs	■					
Pickles							
bread and butter	1 oz	■					
dill	1 oz	■					
Pie							
Apple (McDonald's)	1 pie			■			
Dutch Apple Crumb (Mrs. Smith's)	1/8 pie			■			
Pumpkin Custard (Mrs. Smith's)	1/8 pie			■			

TIP

Freezing does not noticeably raise AGE levels, so don't hesitate to include frozen fruits in your diet. To reduce your intake of added sugar, choose a product that has been prepared without any added sugar or syrup.

FOOD	Portion Size	Very Low	Low	Medium	High	Very High	Highest
Pineapple							
baked	3.5 oz	■	■				
grilled	3.5 oz	■	■				

FOOD	Portion Size	Very Low 100 kU or less	Low 100–500 kU	Medium 501–1,000 kU	High 1,001–3,000 kU	Very High 3,001–5,000 kU	Highest 5,000–12,000 kU
raw	3.5 oz	■					
Pink beans							
boiled	3.5 oz		■				
canned, unheated	3.5 oz		■				
raw	3.5 oz	■	■				
Pinot grigio wine (white)	8 oz	■					
Pinot noir wine (red)	8 oz	■					
Pinto beans							
boiled	3.5 oz		■				
canned, unheated	3.5 oz		■				
raw	3.5 oz	■	■				
Pita bread	2 oz	■					
Pizza, thin crust							
w/mozzarella	3.5 oz						■
w/part-skim mozzarella	3.5 oz				■	■	
w/part-skim mozzarella added during last minute	3.5 oz				■		
Plantain							
baked	3.5 oz	■	■				
grilled	3.5 oz	■	■				
pan-cooked w/cooking spray	3.5 oz	■	■				
raw	3.5 oz	■					
Plantain chips	1 oz		■				

FOOD	Portion Size	Very Low 100 kU or less	Low 100–500 kU	Medium 501–1,000 kU	High 1,001–3,000 kU	Very High 3,001–5,000 kU	Highest 5,000–12,000 kU
Plum							
baked	3.5 oz	■	■				
grilled	3.5 oz	■	■				
poached	3.5 oz	■					
raw	3.5 oz	■					
Pomegranate seeds	3.5 oz	■					
Pop tart							
microwaved	1 tart		■				
not heated	1 tart	■					
toasted	1 tart		■				
Popcorn							
air popped, w/butter	1 oz	■					
microwaved, fat-free	1 oz	■					
Porcini mushrooms							
baked	3.5 oz	■	■				
boiled	3.5 oz	■					
broiled	3.5 oz	■	■				
grilled	3.5 oz	■	■				
raw	3.5 oz	■					
roasted	3.5 oz	■	■				
sautéed w/cooking spray	3.5 oz	■	■				
steamed	3.5 oz	■					
stir-fried w/cooking spray	3.5 oz	■	■				

FOOD	Portion Size	Very Low 100 kU or less	Low 100–500 kU	Medium 501–1,000 kU	High 1,001–3,000 kU	Very High 3,001–5,000 kU	Highest 5,000–12,000 kU
Pork chop							
marinated w/vinegar, barbecued	3 oz				■	■	
marinated w/vinegar, raw	3 oz				■		
pan-fried	3 oz					■	
Pork ribs, roasted	3 oz					■	
Pork roast, loin							
oven-roasted	3 oz					■	
visibly lean, oven-braised w/beer	3 oz			■			
visibly lean, raw	3 oz		■				
Pork tenderloin, lightly browned/braised	3 oz				■		
Portobello mushrooms							
baked	3.5 oz	■	■				
boiled	3.5 oz	■					
broiled	3.5 oz	■	■				
grilled	3.5 oz	■	■				
raw	3.5 oz	■					
roasted	3.5 oz	■	■				
sautéed w/cooking spray	3.5 oz	■	■				
steamed	3.5 oz	■					
stir-fried w/cooking spray	3.5 oz	■	■				
Potato, sweet							
baked	3.5 oz	■	■				

FOOD	Portion Size	Very Low 100 kU or less	Low 100–500 kU	Medium 501–1,000 kU	High 1,001–3,000 kU	Very High 3,001–5,000 kU	Highest 5,000–12,000 kU
boiled	3.5 oz	■					
roasted	3.5 oz	■	■				
steamed	3.5 oz	■					
Potato, white							
baked	3.5 oz	■	■				
boiled	3.5 oz	■					
roasted	3.5 oz	■	■				
steamed	3.5 oz	■					
Potato, white, French fries, cooked in corn oil	3.5 oz			■			
Potato, white, French fries (fast food)							
small	2.5 oz			■	■		
medium	4 oz				■		
large	6 oz				■	■	
Potato, white, hash browns (fast food)	1 hash brown	■	■				
Potato chips							
baked	1 oz		■				
regular	1 oz			■			
Potato salad, lentil	3.5 oz		■				
Pretzels	1 oz		■	■			
Prunes, pitted							
dried	1 oz	■					
stewed	1 oz	■					

FOOD	Portion Size	Very Low 100 kU or less	Low 100–500 kU	Medium 501–1,000 kU	High 1,001–3,000 kU	Very High 3,001–5,000 kU	Highest 5,000–12,000 kU
Pudding, instant, all flavors							
fat-free, sugar-free	1/2 cup	■					
w/skim milk	1/2 cup	■					
Pudding, snack pack, all flavors	1/2 cup	■					
Puffed corn cereal	1 cup	■					
Puffed wheat cereal	1 cup	■					
Pumpkin							
baked	3.5 oz	■	■				
boiled	3.5 oz	■					
raw	3.5 oz	■					
roasted	3.5 oz	■	■				
sautéed w/cooking spray	3.5 oz	■	■				
steamed	3.5 oz	■					
Pumpkin Custard Pie (Mrs. Smith's)	1/8 pie			■			
Pumpkin seeds, raw, hulled	1 oz			■			
Quarter-pound cheese-burger, double (fast food)	1 sand-wich						■
Quince							
cooked	3.5 oz	■					
raw	3.5 oz	■					
Quinoa	3.5 oz	■					
Radicchio	3.5 oz	■					

FOOD	Portion Size	Very Low 100 kU or less	Low 100–500 kU	Medium 501–1,000 kU	High 1,001–3,000 kU	Very High 3,001–5,000 kU	Highest 5,000–12,000 kU
Radish							
grilled	3.5 oz	■	■				
raw	3.5 oz	■					
roasted	3.5 oz	■	■				
Raisinets candy	1.5 oz	■					
Raisins							
cooked	1 oz	■					
dried	1 oz	■					

TIP

Keep the amount of AGEs in vegetables low by going easy on added fats. A good tip is to add just a drizzle of extra-virgin olive oil instead of drenching your dish with oil, butter, or cheese sauce.

FOOD	Portion Size	Very Low	Low	Medium	High	Very High	Highest
Ramps (wild leeks)							
baked	3.5 oz	■	■				
boiled	3.5 oz	■					
broiled	3.5 oz	■	■				
grilled	3.5 oz	■	■				
raw	3.5 oz	■					
roasted	3.5 oz	■	■				
sautéed w/cooking spray	3.5 oz	■	■				
steamed	3.5 oz	■					
stir-fried w/cooking spray	3.5 oz	■	■				

FOOD	Portion Size	Very Low 100 kU or less	Low 100–500 kU	Medium 501–1,000 kU	High 1,001–3,000 kU	Very High 3,001–5,000 kU	Highest 5,000–12,000 kU
Rapini (broccoli rabe)							
baked	3.5 oz	■	■				
boiled	3.5 oz	■					
raw	3.5 oz	■					
sautéed w/cooking spray	3.5 oz	■	■				
steamed	3.5 oz	■					
stir-fried w/cooking spray	3.5 oz	■	■				
Raspberries							
cooked	3.5 oz	■					
raw	3.5 oz	■					
Red wine vinegar	1 Tbs	■					
Resource nutrition drink	8 oz		■				
Ribs, pork, roasted	3 oz					■	
Rice, all varieties	3.5 oz	■					
Rice cake, corn flavored	1 oz	■					
Rice crunch cracker	1 oz		■				
Rice Krispies cereal	1 cup			■			
Rice Krispies Treat bar	1 bar		■	■			
Rice vinegar	1 Tbs	■					
Ricotta cheese, part-skim	1 oz			■			
Roast beef	3 oz						■
Rocket lettuce (arugula)	3.5 oz	■					
Roll, sweet, cinnamon swirl	2.5 oz			■			

FOOD	Portion Size	Very Low 100 kU or less	Low 100–500 kU	Medium 501–1,000 kU	High 1,001–3,000 kU	Very High 3,001–5,000 kU	Highest 5,000–12,000 kU
Roll, dinner	1 oz	■					
Romaine lettuce (cos)	3.5 oz	■					
Rum	1.5 oz	■					
Rum, spiced	1.5 oz	■					
Rutabaga (swede)							
baked	3.5 oz	■	■				
boiled	3.5 oz	■					
braised	3.5 oz	■					
raw	3.5 oz	■					
roasted	3.5 oz	■	■				
sautéed w/cooking spray	3.5 oz	■	■				
steamed	3.5 oz	■					
stir-fried w/cooking spray	3.5 oz	■	■				
Rye whiskey	1.5 oz	■					
Safflower oil	1 Tbs		■	■			
Salad							
Italian pasta	3.5 oz			■			
lentil potato	3.5 oz		■				
tuna pasta	3.5 oz		■				
Salad dressing							
blue cheese	1 Tbs	■	■				
Caesar	1 Tbs		■				
French	1 Tbs	■	■				
French, lite	1 Tbs	■					

FOOD	Portion Size	Very Low 100 kU or less	Low 100–500 kU	Medium 501–1,000 kU	High 1,001–3,000 kU	Very High 3,001–5,000 kU	Highest 5,000–12,000 kU
Italian	1 Tbs	■	■				
Italian, lite	1 Tbs	■					
thousand island	1 Tbs	■	■				

TIP

Although sausages that are fermented and air-dried (such as salami) and boiled meats (such as corned beef) appear to be relatively low in AGEs, they should be limited due to their high amounts of salt, nitrates, and other questionable ingredients. The regular consumption of processed meats has been linked to cancer.

FOOD	Portion Size	Very Low 100 kU or less	Low 100–500 kU	Medium 501–1,000 kU	High 1,001–3,000 kU	Very High 3,001–5,000 kU	Highest 5,000–12,000 kU
Salami, beef kosher	3 oz			■			
Salmon, canned pink	3 oz			■			
Salmon fillet							
boiled	3 oz			■	■		
broiled	3 oz					■	
microwaved	3 oz			■			
pan-fried	3 oz				■	■	
poached	3 oz			■	■		
raw	3 oz		■				
smoked	3 oz			■			
Saltine cracker	1 oz		■				
Sandwich							
bacon, egg & cheese biscuit (fast food)	1 sandwich					■	
cheese melt, open faced	3.5 oz						■

FOOD	Portion Size	Very Low 100 kU or less	Low 100–500 kU	Medium 501–1,000 kU	High 1,001–3,000 kU	Very High 3,001–5,000 kU	Highest 5,000–12,000 kU
cheeseburger (fast food)	1 sandwich					■	
cheeseburger, quarter-pound, double (fast food)	1 sandwich						■
crispy chicken (fast food)	1 sandwich						■
fried fish (fast food)	1 sandwich						■
grilled chicken (fast food)	1 sandwich						■
toasted cheese	3.5 oz					■	
Sandwich, cracker (club crackers w/cheddar)	1 oz			■			
Sausage, Italian							
barbecued	3 oz					■	
raw	3 oz				■		
Sausage, Italian chicken, 96% lean							
pan-fried	3 oz			■	■		
raw	3 oz			■			
Sausage, vegetarian, pan-fried w/cooking spray	2 oz			■			
Sausage links							
beef and pork, pan-fried w/cooking spray	3 oz					■	■
pork, microwaved	3 oz					■	■
Scallion (green onion)							
baked	3.5 oz	■	■				

FOOD	Portion Size	Very Low 100 kU or less	Low 100–500 kU	Medium 501–1,000 kU	High 1,001–3,000 kU	Very High 3,001–5,000 kU	Highest 5,000–12,000 kU
boiled	3.5 oz	■					
broiled	3.5 oz	■	■				
grilled	3.5 oz	■	■				
raw	3.5 oz	■					
roasted	3.5 oz	■	■				
sautéed w/cooking spray	3.5 oz	■	■				
steamed	3.5 oz	■					
stir-fried w/cooking spray	3.5 oz	■	■				
Scone	2.5 oz			■			
Scotch whiskey	1.5 oz	■					
Scrambled egg							
w/butter	1 large		■				
w/cooking spray	1 large	■					
w/corn oil	1 large	■					
w/margarine	1 large	■					
w/olive oil	1 large	■					
Scrod, broiled	3 oz		■	■			

TIP

When preparing high-AGE foods such as beef, poultry, and fish, use AGE-less cooking techniques such as steaming, poaching, stewing, and braising. These moist-heat methods minimize the formation of additional AGEs.

Seafood/Fish. ***See* individual varieties.**

FOOD	Portion Size	Very Low	Low	Medium	High	Very High	Highest
Seeds, pomegranate	3.5 oz	■					

FOOD	Portion Size	Very Low 100 kU or less	Low 100–500 kU	Medium 501–1,000 kU	High 1,001–3,000 kU	Very High 3,001–5,000 kU	Highest 5,000–12,000 kU
Seeds, pumpkin, hulled, raw	1 oz		■	■			
Seeds, sunflower, hulled							
raw	1 oz			■			
roasted and salted	1 oz				■		
Sesame oil	1 Tbs		■				
Sesame oil, toasted	1 Tbs					■	
Shiitake mushrooms							
baked	3.5 oz	■	■				
boiled	3.5 oz	■					
broiled	3.5 oz	■	■				
grilled	3.5 oz	■	■				
raw	3.5 oz	■					
roasted	3.5 oz	■	■				
sautéed w/cooking spray	3.5 oz	■	■				
steamed	3.5 oz	■					
stir-fried w/cooking spray	3.5 oz	■	■				
Shrimp							
breaded, fried	3 oz					■	
marinated and barbecued	3 oz				■		
marinated w/lite balsamic dressing, broiled	3 oz			■			
raw	3 oz		■				
simmered in tomato/white wine sauce	3 oz		■				

FOOD	Portion Size	Very Low 100 kU or less	Low 100–500 kU	Medium 501–1,000 kU	High 1,001–3,000 kU	Very High 3,001–5,000 kU	Highest 5,000–12,000 kU
Snack bar							
Granola, Chocolate Chunk (Quaker)	1 bar		■				
Granola, Peanut Butter/ Chocolate Chip (Quaker)	1 bar			■			
Nutrigrain, Apple Cinnamon	1 bar			■			
Rice Krispies Treat	1 bar		■	■			
Snap peas							
boiled	3.5 oz	■					
raw	3.5 oz	■					
sautéed w/cooking spray	3.5 oz	■	■				
steamed	3.5 oz	■					
stir-fried w/cooking spray	3.5 oz	■	■				
Snickers candy bar	1.5 oz		■				
Snow peas							
boiled	3.5 oz	■					
raw	3.5 oz	■					
sautéed w/cooking spray	3.5 oz	■	■				
steamed	3.5 oz	■					
stir-fried w/cooking spray	3.5 oz	■	■				
Sorbet, fruit	1/2 cup	■					
Soufflé, spinach	3.5 oz			■			
Soup							
beef bouillon	1 cup	■					

FOOD	Portion Size	Very Low 100 kU or less	Low 100–500 kU	Medium 501–1,000 kU	High 1,001–3,000 kU	Very High 3,001–5,000 kU	Highest 5,000–12,000 kU
chicken bouillon	1 cup	■					
chicken broth	1 cup	■					
chicken noodle	1 cup	■					
couscous and lentil	1 cup	■					
cream of celery, low-fat	1 cup		■				
lentil, vegetarian	1 cup		■				
summer vegetable	1 cup	■					
vegetable broth	1 cup	■					

TIP

To keep your AGEs in check, replace meat with plant-based meat alternatives often. Vegetarian bacon, burgers, sausages, and crumbles are all much lower in AGEs than their meat counterparts. Read the labels when choosing these products, though, since some of them are high in sodium and other ingredients that you may wish to avoid.

Soy burger (Boca Burger)							
microwaved	1 burger	■					
oven-baked	1 burger	■	■				
pan-cooked w/cooking spray	1 burger	■					
pan-cooked w/olive oil	1 burger	■	■				
Soy sauce	1 Tbs	■					
Soybeans, roasted and salted	1 oz		■	■			
Soymilk	1 cup	■					

FOOD	Portion Size	Very Low 100 kU or less	Low 100–500 kU	Medium 501–1,000 kU	High 1,001–3,000 kU	Very High 3,001–5,000 kU	Highest 5,000–12,000 kU
Spaghetti squash							
baked	3.5 oz	■	■				
boiled	3.5 oz	■					
roasted	3.5 oz	■	■				
sautéed w/cooking spray	3.5 oz	■	■				
steamed	3.5 oz	■					
Spelt	3.5 oz	■					
Spinach							
boiled	3.5 oz	■					
raw	3.5 oz	■					
sautéed w/cooking spray	3.5 oz	■	■				
steamed	3.5 oz	■					
stir-fried w/cooking spray	3.5 oz	■	■				
Spinach soufflé	3.5 oz			■			
Split peas							
boiled	3.5 oz		■				
canned, unheated	3.5 oz		■				
raw	3.5 oz	■	■				
Sprite							
diet	8 oz	■					
regular	8 oz	■					
Squash, acorn							
baked	3.5 oz	■	■				
boiled	3.5 oz	■					

FOOD	Portion Size	Very Low 100 kU or less	Low 100–500 kU	Medium 501–1,000 kU	High 1,001–3,000 kU	Very High 3,001–5,000 kU	Highest 5,000–12,000 kU
broiled	3.5 oz	■	■				
grilled	3.5 oz	■	■				
raw	3.5 oz	■					
roasted	3.5 oz	■	■				
steamed	3.5 oz	■					
Squash, butternut							
baked	3.5 oz	■	■				
boiled	3.5 oz	■					
broiled	3.5 oz	■	■				
grilled	3.5 oz	■	■				
raw	3.5 oz	■					
roasted	3.5 oz	■	■				
steamed	3.5 oz	■					
Squash, spaghetti							
baked	3.5 oz	■	■				
boiled	3.5 oz	■					
roasted	3.5 oz	■	■				
sautéed w/cooking spray	3.5 oz	■	■				
steamed	3.5 oz	■					
Star fruit	3.5 oz	■					
Strawberries							
cooked	3.5 oz	■					
raw	3.5 oz	■					

FOOD	Portion Size	Very Low 100 kU or less	Low 100–500 kU	Medium 501–1,000 kU	High 1,001–3,000 kU	Very High 3,001–5,000 kU	Highest 5,000–12,000 kU
Steak, beef							
broiled	3 oz						■
grilled (nonstick grill)	3 oz						■
microwaved	3 oz				■		
pan-fried	3 oz						■
raw	3 oz			■			
stir-fried (strips)	3 oz						■
Steak, beef, top sirloin, trimmed							
grilled (nonstick grill), rare	3 oz			■			
grilled (nonstick grill), medium	3 oz				■		
grilled (nonstick grill), well done	3 oz				■		
raw	3 oz		■	■			
Sugar, white granulated	1 tsp	■					
Sugar substitute, aspartame	1 tsp	■					

TIP

Although sugar and high-sugar sweeteners are low in AGEs, their use should be limited. When sugar is added to foods and heated—when cookies are baked, for instance—the sugar can react with fats and proteins to make AGEs. Plus, a high-sugar diet can contribute to obesity, insulin resistance, and eventually, diabetes.

FOOD	Portion Size	Very Low	Low	Medium	High	Very High	Highest
Summer vegetable soup	1 cup	■					
Sunflower oil	1 Tbs			■			

FOOD	Portion Size	Very Low 100 kU or less	Low 100–500 kU	Medium 501–1,000 kU	High 1,001–3,000 kU	Very High 3,001–5,000 kU	Highest 5,000–12,000 kU
Sunflower seeds, hulled							
raw	1 oz			■			
roasted and salted	1 oz				■		
Swede (rutabaga)							
baked	3.5 oz	■	■				
boiled	3.5 oz	■					
braised	3.5 oz	■					
raw	3.5 oz	■					
roasted	3.5 oz	■	■				
sautéed w/cooking spray	3.5 oz	■	■				
steamed	3.5 oz	■					
stir-fried w/cooking spray	3.5 oz	■	■				
Sweet potato							
baked	3.5 oz	■	■				
boiled	3.5 oz	■					
roasted	3.5 oz	■	■				
steamed	3.5 oz	■					
Sweet roll, cinnamon swirl	2.5 oz			■			
Swiss chard							
boiled	3.5 oz	■					
raw	3.5 oz	■					
sautéed w/cooking spray	3.5 oz	■	■				
steamed	3.5 oz	■					
stir-fried w/cooking spray	3.5 oz	■	■				

FOOD	Portion Size	Very Low 100 kU or less	Low 100–500 kU	Medium 501–1,000 kU	High 1,001–3,000 kU	Very High 3,001–5,000 kU	Highest 5,000–12,000 kU
Swiss cheese							
reduced-fat	1 oz			■	■		
regular	1 oz				■		
Syrup							
caramel, sugar-free	1 Tbs	■					
dark corn	1 Tbs	■					
pancake	1 Tbs	■					
pancake, lite	1 Tbs	■					
Tangerine	3.5 oz	■					
Taramosalata caviar spread	3.5 oz			■			
Tartar sauce	1 Tbs	■	■				
Tatsoi salad greens	3.5 oz	■					
Tea							
decaf	8 oz	■					
flavored	8 oz	■					
herbal	8 oz	■					
regular	8 oz	■					
Tequila	1.5 oz	■					
Thousand Island salad dressing	1 Tbs	■	■				
Timbale, broccoli	3.5 oz		■				
Toast, French, frozen (Aunt Jemima)							
in toaster oven	1 slice		■				

FOOD	Portion Size	Very Low	Low	Medium	High	Very High	Highest
		100 kU or less	100–500 kU	501–1,000 kU	1,001–3,000 kU	3,001–5,000 kU	5,000–12,000 kU
microwaved	1 slice		■				
not heated	1 slice	■	■				
Toast, French, whole grain, low-fat	1 slice	■	■				
Toast, melba	1 oz		■				
Toasted wheat cracker	1 oz		■				

TIP

Eat tofu raw, steamed, or simmered in soup. Broiling, grilling, or sautéing tofu causes a dramatic rise in AGEs.

FOOD	Portion Size	Very Low	Low	Medium	High	Very High	Highest
Tofu							
broiled	3 oz					■	
raw	3 oz			■			
sautéed	3 oz					■	
Tofu, soft							
boiled	3 oz			■			
raw	3 oz		■				
Tomato							
baked	3.5 oz	■	■				
boiled	3.5 oz	■					
broiled	3.5 oz	■	■				
grilled	3.5 oz	■	■				
raw	3.5 oz	■					
roasted	3.5 oz	■	■				
steamed	3.5 oz	■					

FOOD	Portion Size	Very Low 100 kU or less	Low 100–500 kU	Medium 501–1,000 kU	High 1,001–3,000 kU	Very High 3,001–5,000 kU	Highest 5,000–12,000 kU
Tomato sauce	3.5 oz	■					
Total cereal, wheat and brown rice	1 cup	■					
Trout							
baked	3 oz				■		
raw	3 oz			■			
Trumpet mushrooms							
baked	3.5 oz	■	■				
boiled	3.5 oz	■					
broiled	3.5 oz	■	■				
grilled	3.5 oz	■	■				
raw	3.5 oz	■					
roasted	3.5 oz	■	■				
sautéed w/cooking spray	3.5 oz	■	■				
steamed	3.5 oz	■					
stir-fried w/cooking spray	3.5 oz	■	■				
Tuna							
baked	3 oz			■			
broiled w/vinaigrette dressing	3 oz					■	
Tuna, canned							
chunk light in water	3 oz		■				
white albacore in oil	3 oz				■		
Tuna casserole	3.5 oz		■				

FOOD	Portion Size	Very Low 100 kU or less	Low 100–500 kU	Medium 501–1,000 kU	High 1,001–3,000 kU	Very High 3,001–5,000 kU	Highest 5,000–12,000 kU
Tuna loaf, w/chunk light, baked	3 oz			■			
Tuna patty, w/chunk light, broiled	3 oz			■			

> **TIP**
>
> A higher fat content means higher AGEs, so buy lean cuts of meat and trim away any external fat. When shopping for ground meat, look for a product that is at least 93-percent lean.

FOOD	Portion Size	Very Low	Low	Medium	High	Very High	Highest
Turkey, ground							
grilled	3 oz						■
raw	3 oz					■	
Turkey, ground, 94% lean							
pan-cooked w/cooking spray	3 oz			■	■		
raw	3 oz			■			
Turkey breast, skinless							
oven braised	3 oz			■	■		
raw	3 oz		■				
roasted	3 oz					■	
smoked, seared	3 oz						■
Turkey burger							
broiled	3 oz					■	
pan-fried	3 oz						■
Turkey burger, 94% lean							
pan-fried	3 oz				■		

FOOD	Portion Size	Very Low 100 kU or less	Low 100–500 kU	Medium 501–1,000 kU	High 1,001–3,000 kU	Very High 3,001–5,000 kU	Highest 5,000–12,000 kU
Turnip							
baked	3.5 oz	■	■				
boiled	3.5 oz	■					
raw	3.5 oz	■					
roasted	3.5 oz	■	■				
sautéed w/cooking spray	3.5 oz	■	■				
steamed	3.5 oz	■					
stir-fried w/cooking spray	3.5 oz	■	■				
Vanilla wafer cookie	1 oz		■				
Veal, stewed	3 oz				■		
Vegetable broth	1 cup	■					
Vegetable juice	8 oz	■					
Vegetable soup, summer	1 cup	■					
Vegetables. *See* individual varieties.							
Veggie burger, California (Amy's)							
microwaved	1 burger	■					
oven-baked	1 burger		■				
pan-cooked w/cooking spray	1 burger	■	■				
pan-cooked w/olive oil	1 burger		■				
Vinegar							
apple cider	1 Tbs	■					
balsamic	1 Tbs	■					
red wine	1 Tbs	■					

FOOD	Portion Size	Very Low 100 kU or less	Low 100–500 kU	Medium 501–1,000 kU	High 1,001–3,000 kU	Very High 3,001–5,000 kU	Highest 5,000–12,000 kU
rice	1 Tbs	■					
white	1 Tbs	■					
white wine	1 Tbs	■					
Vodka	1.5 oz	■					
Waffle, frozen, toasted	1 waffle			■			
Walnuts, roasted	1 oz				■		
Watercress (cress)	3.5 oz	■					
Watermelon							
grilled	3.5 oz	■	■				
raw	3.5 oz	■					
Wehani rice	3.5 oz	■					
Wheat cracker							
plain	1 oz		■				
toasted	1 oz		■				
Whiskey	1.5 oz	■					
White button mushrooms							
baked	3.5 oz	■	■				
boiled	3.5 oz	■					
broiled	3.5 oz	■	■				
grilled	3.5 oz	■	■				
raw	3.5 oz	■					
roasted	3.5 oz	■	■				
sautéed w/cooking spray	3.5 oz	■	■				
steamed	3.5 oz	■					

FOOD	Portion Size	Very Low 100 kU or less	Low 100–500 kU	Medium 501–1,000 kU	High 1,001–3,000 kU	Very High 3,001–5,000 kU	Highest 5,000–12,000 kU
stir-fried w/cooking spray	3.5 oz	■	■				
White rice							
quick-cooking	3.5 oz	■					
regular	3.5 oz	■					
White vinegar	1 Tbs	■					
White wine vinegar	1 Tbs	■					
Whiting, breaded, oven-fried	3 oz						■
Wild leeks (ramps)							
baked	3.5 oz	■	■				
boiled	3.5 oz	■					
broiled	3.5 oz	■	■				
grilled	3.5 oz	■	■				
raw	3.5 oz	■					
roasted	3.5 oz	■	■				
sautéed w/cooking spray	3.5 oz	■	■				
steamed	3.5 oz	■					
stir-fried w/cooking spray	3.5 oz	■	■				
Wild rice	3.5 oz	■					
Wine							
pinot grigio (white)	8 oz	■					
pinot noir (red)	8 oz	■					
Witloof (Belgian endive, endive)	3.5 oz	■					

FOOD	Portion Size	Very Low 100 kU or less	Low 100–500 kU	Medium 501–1,000 kU	High 1,001–3,000 kU	Very High 3,001–5,000 kU	Highest 5,000–12,000 kU
Won ton, pork, fried	3.5 oz				■		
Yogurt							
plain	1 cup	■					
vanilla	1 cup	■					
w/fruit	1 cup	■					

TIP

Make yogurt—a high-nutrient, low-AGE food—part of your diet. For everyday use, choose low-fat or nonfat products, as they will also be lower in calories and saturated fat. For the greatest health benefits, choose plain yogurt and add fruit and only a small amount of sweetener.

FOOD	Portion Size	Very Low 100 kU or less	Low 100–500 kU	Medium 501–1,000 kU	High 1,001–3,000 kU	Very High 3,001–5,000 kU	Highest 5,000–12,000 kU
Ziti, baked	3.5 oz				■		
Zucchini (courgette)							
baked	3.5 oz	■	■				
boiled	3.5 oz	■					
broiled	3.5 oz	■	■				
grilled	3.5 oz	■	■				
raw	3.5 oz	■					
roasted	3.5 oz	■	■				
sautéed w/cooking spray	3.5 oz	■	■				
steamed	3.5 oz	■					
stir-fried w/cooking spray	3.5 oz	■	■				

Food Listing by Category

FOOD	Portion Size	Very Low 100 kU or less	Low 100–500 kU	Medium 501–1,000 kU	High 1,001–3,000 kU	Very High 3,001–5,000 kU	Highest 5,000–12,000 kU
BEANS/LEGUMES							
Black beans							
boiled	3.5 oz		■				
canned, unheated	3.5 oz		■				
raw	3.5 oz	■	■				
Black-eyed peas							
boiled	3.5 oz		■				
canned, unheated	3.5 oz		■				
raw	3.5 oz	■	■				
Cannellini beans							
boiled	3.5 oz		■				
canned, unheated	3.5 oz		■				
raw	3.5 oz	■	■				

TIP

To trim AGEs from your diet, enjoy legumes—beans, peas, and lentils—as often as possible. In addition to being low in AGEs, legumes are inexpensive, super-nutritious, and highly versatile.

FOOD	Portion Size	Very Low	Low	Medium	High	Very High	Highest
Chickpeas							
boiled	3.5 oz		■				
canned, unheated	3.5 oz		■				
raw	3.5 oz	■	■				
Edamame							
boiled	3.5 oz	■					
steamed	3.5 oz	■					

FOOD	Portion Size	Very Low 100 kU or less	Low 100–500 kU	Medium 501–1,000 kU	High 1,001–3,000 kU	Very High 3,001–5,000 kU	Highest 5,000–12,000 kU
Fava beans							
boiled	3.5 oz		■				
raw	3.5 oz	■	■				
Garbanzo beans. *See* Chickpeas.							
Great Northern beans							
boiled	3.5 oz		■				
canned, unheated	3.5 oz		■				
raw	3.5 oz	■	■				
Kidney beans, red							
boiled	3.5 oz		■				
canned, unheated	3.5 oz		■				
raw	3.5 oz	■	■				
Lentils							
boiled	3.5 oz		■				
canned, unheated	3.5 oz		■				
raw	3.5 oz	■	■				
Lima beans							
boiled	3.5 oz		■				
canned, unheated	3.5 oz		■				
raw	3.5 oz	■	■				
Navy beans							
boiled	3.5 oz		■				
canned, unheated	3.5 oz		■				
raw	3.5 oz	■	■				

FOOD	Portion Size	Very Low 100 kU or less	Low 100–500 kU	Medium 501–1,000 kU	High 1,001–3,000 kU	Very High 3,001–5,000 kU	Highest 5,000–12,000 kU
Peanuts							
cocktail	1 oz				■		
dry roasted, unsalted	1 oz				■		
roasted in shell, salted	1 oz			■	■		
Peas, fresh							
boiled	3.5 oz	■					
canned, unheated	3.5 oz	■					
raw	3.5 oz	■					
sautéed w/cooking spray	3.5 oz	■	■				
steamed	3.5 oz	■					
stir-fried w/cooking spray	3.5 oz	■	■				
Pink beans							
boiled	3.5 oz		■				
canned, unheated	3.5 oz		■				
raw	3.5 oz	■	■				
Pinto beans							
boiled	3.5 oz		■				
canned, unheated	3.5 oz		■				
raw	3.5 oz	■	■				
Snap peas							
boiled	3.5 oz	■					
raw	3.5 oz	■					
sautéed w/cooking spray	3.5 oz	■	■				
steamed	3.5 oz	■					

FOOD	Portion Size	Very Low 100 kU or less	Low 100–500 kU	Medium 501–1,000 kU	High 1,001–3,000 kU	Very High 3,001–5,000 kU	Highest 5,000–12,000 kU
stir-fried w/cooking spray	3.5 oz	■	■				
Snow peas							
boiled	3.5 oz	■					
raw	3.5 oz	■					
sautéed w/cooking spray	3.5 oz	■	■				
steamed	3.5 oz	■					
stir-fried w/cooking spray	3.5 oz	■	■				
Soybeans, roasted and salted	1 oz		■	■			
Split peas							
boiled	3.5 oz		■				
canned, unheated	3.5 oz		■				
raw	3.5 oz	■	■				
BEEF/BEEF DISHES							
Bologna	3 oz				■		
Corned beef, low-fat	3 oz			■			
Corned beef hash, canned							
microwaved	3.5 oz				■		
pan-heated	3.5 oz				■		
unheated	3.5 oz			■	■		
Frankfurter							
boiled	3 oz					■	■
broiled	3 oz						■

FOOD	Portion Size	Very Low 100 kU or less	Low 100–500 kU	Medium 501–1,000 kU	High 1,001–3,000 kU	Very High 3,001–5,000 kU	Highest 5,000–12,000 kU
Ground beef							
80% lean, pan-browned	3 oz					■	
91% lean, grass-fed, pan-browned	3 oz			■			
91% lean, grass-fed, raw	3 oz		■				
93% lean, pan-browned	3 oz			■	■		
93% lean, raw	3 oz			■			
Hamburger patty (fast food)	3 oz					■	

TIP

When buying beef, choose organic grass-fed products whenever possible. Meat from grass-fed animals is lower in AGEs than meat from conventionally raised animals.

FOOD	Portion Size	Very Low	Low	Medium	High	Very High	Highest
Hamburger patty, 93% lean							
grilled (nonstick grill)	3 oz				■		
pan-cooked	3 oz				■		
Hot dog. *See* Frankfurter.							
Meatball							
simmered in broth	3 oz					■	
93% lean, simmered in tomato sauce	3 oz				■		
Meatloaf							
oven-baked	3 oz				■		
93% lean, oven-baked	3 oz			■			
Roast beef	3 oz						■

FOOD	Portion Size	Very Low 100 kU or less	Low 100–500 kU	Medium 501–1,000 kU	High 1,001–3,000 kU	Very High 3,001–5,000 kU	Highest 5,000–12,000 kU
Salami, kosher	3 oz			■			
Sausage links							
beef and pork, pan-fried w/cooking spray	3 oz					■	■
Shoulder cut							
raw	3 oz			■			
stewed	3 oz				■		
Steak							
broiled	3 oz						■
grilled (nonstick grill)	3 oz						■
microwaved	3 oz				■		
pan-fried	3 oz						■
raw	3 oz			■			
stir-fried (strips)	3 oz						■
Steak, top sirloin, trimmed							
grilled (nonstick grill), rare	3 oz			■			
grilled (nonstick grill), medium	3 oz				■		
grilled (nonstick grill), well done	3 oz				■		
raw	3 oz		■	■			
Top round chunks							
raw	3 oz		■	■			
stewed	3 oz			■			

FOOD	Portion Size	Very Low 100 kU or less	Low 100–500 kU	Medium 501–1,000 kU	High 1,001–3,000 kU	Very High 3,001–5,000 kU	Highest 5,000–12,000 kU
Top round roast							
oven-braised	3 oz				■		
pressure-cooked	3 oz				■		
raw	3 oz		■	■			
BEVERAGES							
Apple juice	8 oz	■					
Beer	9 oz	■					
Coca Cola							
classic	8 oz	■					
diet	8 oz	■					
Cocoa (Swiss Miss)							
regular	1 cup			■			
sugar-free	1 cup		■	■			
Coconut milk	1/3 cup		■				
Coffee							
instant	1 cup	■					
instant, decaf	1 cup	■					
regular	1 cup	■					
Spanish	1 cup	■					
w/milk	1 cup	■					
w/sugar	1 cup	■					
Coke. ***See*** **Coca Cola.**							
Cranberry juice	8 oz	■					
Enfamil infant formula	2 Tbs		■				

FOOD	Portion Size	Very Low 100 kU or less	Low 100–500 kU	Medium 501–1,000 kU	High 1,001–3,000 kU	Very High 3,001–5,000 kU	Highest 5,000–12,000 kU
Ensure Plus nutrition drink	8 oz	■					
Gin	1.5 oz	■					
Glucerna nutrition drink	8 oz		■				
Malta malt beverage	8 oz	■					
Milk							
fat-free	1 cup	■					
fat-free w/vitamins A and D	1 cup	■					
reduced fat	1 cup	■					
soy	1 cup	■					
whole	1 cup	■					
Milk, breast							
fresh	1 oz	■					
frozen	1 oz	■					
Milk, coconut	1/3 cup		■				
Orange juice							
regular	8 oz	■					
w/calcium	8 oz	■					
Pepsi Cola							
diet	8 oz	■					
diet, caffeine-free	8 oz	■					
regular	8 oz	■					
Resource nutrition drink	8 oz		■				
Rum	1.5 oz	■					

FOOD	Portion Size	Very Low 100 kU or less	Low 100–500 kU	Medium 501–1,000 kU	High 1,001–3,000 kU	Very High 3,001–5,000 kU	Highest 5,000–12,000 kU
Rum, spiced	1.5 oz	■					
Rye whiskey	1.5 oz	■					
Scotch whiskey	1.5 oz	■					
Sprite							
diet	8 oz	■					
regular	8 oz	■					
Tea							
decaf	8 oz	■					
flavored	8 oz	■					
herbal	8 oz	■					
regular	8 oz	■					
Tequila	1.5 oz	■					
Vegetable juice	8 oz	■					
Vodka	1.5 oz	■					
Whiskey	1.5 oz	■					
Wine							
red (pinot noir)	8 oz	■					
white (pinot grigio)	8 oz	■					
BREAD							
Bagel							
toasted	2 oz		■				
untoasted	2 oz	■					
Biscuit	2 oz			■			
Breadsticks	1 oz	■					

FOOD	Portion Size	Very Low 100 kU or less	Low 100–500 kU	Medium 501–1,000 kU	High 1,001–3,000 kU	Very High 3,001–5,000 kU	Highest 5,000–12,000 kU
Italian bread							
toasted	2 oz	■					
untoasted	2 oz	■					
Pita bread	2 oz	■					
White bread							
toasted	2 oz	■					
untoasted	2 oz	■					
Whole wheat bread							
toasted	2 oz	■					
untoasted	2 oz	■					
BREAKFAST FOODS. ***See also*** **Cereal; Eggs/Egg Dishes.**							
Bacon, egg & cheese biscuit (fast food)	1 sandwich					■	
Bacon, Egg & Cheese Hot Pocket							
microwaved	1 pocket			■	■		
not heated	1 pocket			■			
oven-baked	1 pocket				■		
Bagel							
toasted	2 oz		■				
untoasted	2 oz	■					
Biscuit	2 oz			■			
Bran muffin	2.5 oz		■				
Croissant, classic butter	2 oz			■			
Danish, cheese	2.5 oz			■			

FOOD	Portion Size	Very Low 100 kU or less	Low 100–500 kU	Medium 501–1,000 kU	High 1,001–3,000 kU	Very High 3,001–5,000 kU	Highest 5,000–12,000 kU
French toast, frozen (Aunt Jemima)							
in toaster oven	1 slice		■				
microwaved	1 slice		■				
not heated	1 slice	■	■				
French toast, whole grain, low-fat	1 slice	■	■				
Hotcakes (McDonald's)	3 hot-cakes		■				
Pancake							
from mix	1 oz		■				
frozen, toasted	1 oz			■			
Scone	2.5 oz			■			
Waffle, frozen, toasted	1 waffle			■			
CAKES/PIES/BAKED GOODS. ***See also*** **Cookies/Crackers.**							
Angel food cake	1 oz	■					
Apple Crumb Pie, Dutch (Mrs. Smith's)				■			
Apple pie (McDonald's)	1 pie			■			
Banana bread, low-fat	2 oz	■	■				
Bran muffin	2.5 oz		■				
Croissant, classic butter	2 oz			■			
Danish, cheese	2.5 oz			■			
Donut							
chocolate iced, cream-filled	2.5 oz			■	■		

FOOD	Portion Size	Very Low 100 kU or less	Low 100–500 kU	Medium 501–1,000 kU	High 1,001–3,000 kU	Very High 3,001–5,000 kU	Highest 5,000–12,000 kU
devil's food cake, glazed	2.5 oz			■	■		
Pumpkin Custard Pie (Mrs. Smith's)	1/8 pie			■			
Scone	2.5 oz			■			
Sweet roll, cinnamon swirl	2.5 oz			■			

TIP

When you want to indulge, choose a relatively low-AGE dessert—a dairy treat such as ice cream or pudding, or a fruit dessert such as sorbet or grilled fruit. When sweeteners are added to other ingredients and heated—when you bake cakes or cookies, for instance—they can react with proteins and fats to form AGEs.

FOOD	Portion Size	Very Low 100 kU or less	Low 100–500 kU	Medium 501–1,000 kU	High 1,001–3,000 kU	Very High 3,001–5,000 kU	Highest 5,000–12,000 kU
CANDY							
Chocolate, Hershey's Special Dark	1.5 oz		■	■			
Ginger, crystallized	2 tsp	■					
M & M's, milk chocolate	1.5 oz			■			
Peanut Butter Cup, Reese's	1.5 oz				■		
Raisinets	1.5 oz	■					
Snickers bar	1.5 oz		■				
CEREAL							
Bran flakes	1 cup	■					
Cinnamon Toast Crunch	1 cup		■				
Corn Flakes	1 cup	■					
Corn Pops	1 cup		■				

FOOD	Portion Size	Very Low 100 kU or less	Low 100–500 kU	Medium 501–1,000 kU	High 1,001–3,000 kU	Very High 3,001–5,000 kU	Highest 5,000–12,000 kU
Cream of Wheat							
plain	3/4 cup		■				
w/honey	3/4 cup		■				
Honey Nut Cheerios	1 cup	■	■				
Fiber One	1 cup		■				
Froot Loops	1 cup	■					
Frosted Flakes	1 cup		■				
Frosted Mini Wheats	1 cup	■					
Granola, Organic Oats & Honey	2/3 cup		■				
Life	1 cup		■				
Oatmeal, traditional and instant							
plain	1 cup	■					
w/honey	1 cup	■					
Puffed corn	1 cup	■					
Puffed wheat	1 cup	■					
Rice Krispies	1 cup			■			
Total, wheat and brown rice	1 cup	■					
CHEESE							
American							
low-fat	1 oz			■	■		
regular	1 oz				■		
Brie	1 oz				■		

FOOD	Portion Size	Very Low 100 kU or less	Low 100–500 kU	Medium 501–1,000 kU	High 1,001–3,000 kU	Very High 3,001–5,000 kU	Highest 5,000–12,000 kU
Cheddar							
regular	1 oz				■		
white, 75% light	1 oz			■	■		
w/2% milk	1 oz			■			
Cottage, 1% fat	1 oz		■				
Cream	1 oz				■		
Feta, Greek, soft	1 oz				■		

TIP

Avoid cheese with labels like "processed cheese," "prepared cheese product," or "cheese food." These products have undergone additional heating, melting, and processing steps that raise their AGE content.

FOOD	Portion Size	Very Low	Low	Medium	High	Very High	Highest
Mozzarella							
fresh	1 oz		■	■			
part-skim	1 oz			■	■		
Parmesan, grated	2 Tbs				■		
Ricotta, part-skim	1 oz			■			
Swiss							
reduced-fat	1 oz			■	■		
regular	1 oz				■		
CHICKEN/CHICKEN DISHES							
Breast, skinless							
boiled	3 oz			■			
breaded, deep-fried	3 oz						■

FOOD	Portion Size	Very Low 100 kU or less	Low 100–500 kU	Medium 501–1,000 kU	High 1,001–3,000 kU	Very High 3,001–5,000 kU	Highest 5,000–12,000 kU
breaded, pan-fried	3 oz						■
broiled	3 oz					■	■
grilled (nonstick grill)	3 oz					■	
marinated w/lemon, grilled (nonstick grill)	3 oz			■			
microwaved	3 oz				■		
oven-baked w/white wine in parchment	3 oz			■			
pan-fried	3 oz					■	
poached	3 oz			■			
raw	3 oz		■				
roasted	3 oz					■	■
simmered	3 oz			■			
in slow-cooker	3 oz			■			
steamed in foil	3 oz			■			
Breast, w/skin							
breaded, oven-fried	3 oz						■
broiled	3 oz						■
roasted	3 oz						■
Breast strips							
stir-fried w/oil	3 oz					■	
stir-fried w/out oil	3 oz				■	■	
Burger, 89% lean							
pan-fried w/cooking spray	3 oz				■		

FOOD	Portion Size	Very Low 100 kU or less	Low 100–500 kU	Medium 501–1,000 kU	High 1,001–3,000 kU	Very High 3,001–5,000 kU	Highest 5,000–12,000 kU
Ground chicken							
89% lean, raw	3 oz		■	■			
dark meat, w/skin, pan-fried	3 oz				■	■	
dark meat, w/skin, raw	3 oz			■	■		
white meat, skinless, pan-fried	3 oz				■		
white meat, skinless, raw	3 oz			■			

TIP

When preparing high-AGE foods such as beef, poultry, and fish, use AGE-less cooking techniques such as steaming, poaching, stewing, and braising. These moist-heat methods minimize the formation of additional AGEs.

FOOD	Portion Size	Very Low 100 kU or less	Low 100–500 kU	Medium 501–1,000 kU	High 1,001–3,000 kU	Very High 3,001–5,000 kU	Highest 5,000–12,000 kU
Kebab, w/skinless breast cubes							
pan-fried	3 oz					■	■
Leg							
skinless, roasted	3 oz					■	
w/skin, roasted	3 oz						■
Loaf, baked	3 oz				■	■	
Nuggets, fried (fast food)	6 nuggets						■
Sandwich							
crispy (fast food)	1 sandwich						■
grilled (fast food)	1 sandwich						■

FOOD	Portion Size	Very Low 100 kU or less	Low 100–500 kU	Medium 501–1,000 kU	High 1,001–3,000 kU	Very High 3,001–5,000 kU	Highest 5,000–12,000 kU
Sausage, Italian, 96% lean							
pan-cooked	3 oz			■	■		
raw	3 oz			■			
Thigh, w/skin, roasted	3 oz						■

COLD CUTS. *See* Luncheon Meats.

TIP

Skip high-sugar condiments like ketchup and sweet barbecue sauce. Although they are low in AGEs, because of their high sugar content, these products can boost AGE levels if used in excess and on a frequent basis.

CONDIMENTS

FOOD	Portion Size	Very Low 100 kU or less	Low 100–500 kU	Medium 501–1,000 kU	High 1,001–3,000 kU	Very High 3,001–5,000 kU	Highest 5,000–12,000 kU
Apple cider vinegar	1 Tbs	■					
Balsamic vinegar	1 Tbs	■					
Ginger, raw, grated	2 tsp	■					
Ketchup	1 Tbs	■					
Mayonnaise							
fat-free	1 Tbs	■					
low-fat	1 Tbs		■				
regular	1 Tbs			■			
Mustard	1 Tbs	■					
Olives, ripe	1 oz			■			
Pickles							
bread and butter	1 oz	■					
dill	1 oz	■					

FOOD	Portion Size	Very Low 100 kU or less	Low 100–500 kU	Medium 501–1,000 kU	High 1,001–3,000 kU	Very High 3,001–5,000 kU	Highest 5,000–12,000 kU
Red wine vinegar	1 Tbs	■					
Rice vinegar	1 Tbs	■					
Soy sauce	1 Tbs	■					
Tartar sauce	1 Tbs	■	■				
Tomato sauce	3.5 oz	■					
White vinegar	1 Tbs	■					
White wine vinegar	1 Tbs	■					
COOKIES/CRACKERS							
Biscotti cookie, vanilla almond	1 oz			■			
Chocolate chip cookie	1 oz			■			
Chocolate graham cracker	1 oz		■				
Fortune cookie	1 oz	■					
Goldfish cracker, cheddar	1 oz			■			
Honey graham cracker	1 oz		■				
Melba toast	1 oz		■				
Meringue cookie	1 oz		■				
Oatmeal raisin cookie	1 oz		■				
Oreo cookie	1 oz			■			
Oyster cracker	1 oz			■			
Rice cake, corn flavored	1 oz	■					
Rice crunch cracker	1 oz		■				
Saltine cracker	1 oz		■				

FOOD	Portion Size	Very Low 100 kU or less	Low 100–500 kU	Medium 501–1,000 kU	High 1,001–3,000 kU	Very High 3,001–5,000 kU	Highest 5,000–12,000 kU
Sandwich cracker (w/cheddar)	1 oz			■			
Toasted wheat cracker	1 oz		■				
Vanilla wafer cookie	1 oz		■				
Wheat cracker	1 oz		■				
DAIRY PRODUCTS							
American cheese							
low-fat	1 oz			■	■		
regular	1 oz				■		
Brie	1 oz				■		
Butter							
browned	1 Tbs				■		
clarified	1 Tbs				■	■	
unsalted	1 Tbs				■		
whipped	1 Tbs				■		
Cheddar cheese							
regular	1 oz				■		
white, 75% light	1 oz			■	■		
w/2% milk	1 oz			■			
Cottage cheese, 1% fat	1 oz		■				
Cream, heavy, ultra-pasteurized	1 Tbs		■				
Cream cheese	1 oz				■		
Feta cheese, Greek, soft	1 oz				■		

FOOD	Portion Size	Very Low 100 kU or less	Low 100–500 kU	Medium 501–1,000 kU	High 1,001–3,000 kU	Very High 3,001–5,000 kU	Highest 5,000–12,000 kU
Ice cream, vanilla	1 cup	■					
Milk							
fat-free	1 cup	■					
fat-free w/vitamins A and D	1 cup	■					
reduced fat	1 cup	■					
soy	1 cup	■					
whole	1 cup	■					

TIP

Nonfat, reduced-fat, and whole milk are all low in AGEs. To trim calories and saturated fat, choose the lower-fat varieties. Save whole milk for coffee or recipes in which you want to add richness. Avoid cream, which contains many more AGEs than milk.

FOOD	Portion Size	Very Low 100 kU or less	Low 100–500 kU	Medium 501–1,000 kU	High 1,001–3,000 kU	Very High 3,001–5,000 kU	Highest 5,000–12,000 kU
Mozzarella cheese							
fresh	1 oz		■	■			
part-skim	1 oz			■	■		
Parmesan cheese, grated	2 Tbs				■		
Ricotta cheese, part-skim	1 oz			■			
Swiss cheese							
reduced-fat	1 oz			■	■		
regular	1 oz				■		
Yogurt							
plain	1 cup	■					
vanilla	1 cup	■					
w/fruit	1 cup	■					

FOOD	Portion Size	Very Low 100 kU or less	Low 100–500 kU	Medium 501–1,000 kU	High 1,001–3,000 kU	Very High 3,001–5,000 kU	Highest 5,000–12,000 kU
DIPS/SPREADS/SAUCES							
Butter							
browned	1 Tbs				■		
clarified	1 Tbs				■	■	
unsalted	1 Tbs				■		
whipped	1 Tbs				■		
Caviar spread, taramosalata	3.5 oz			■			
Coconut cream	1 Tbs	■	■				
Cream cheese	1 oz				■		
Hummus	3.5 oz			■			
Ketchup	1 Tbs	■					
Margarine	1 Tbs			■	■		
Mayonnaise							
fat-free	1 Tbs	■					
low-fat	1 Tbs		■				
regular	1 Tbs			■			
Mustard	1 Tbs	■					
Peanut butter, smooth	2 Tbs				■		
Pesto, with basil	1 Tbs	■					
Soy sauce	1 Tbs	■					
Tartar sauce	1 Tbs	■	■				
Tomato sauce	3.5 oz	■					

FOOD	Portion Size	Very Low 100 kU or less	Low 100–500 kU	Medium 501–1,000 kU	High 1,001–3,000 kU	Very High 3,001–5,000 kU	Highest 5,000–12,000 kU
EGGS/EGG DISHES							
Fried	1 large				■		
Hard boiled							
egg white	1 large	■					
egg yolk	1 large		■				
TIP Enjoy eggs as a high-nutrient, low-AGE source of protein. To keep AGE formation at the lowest possible level, poach your eggs or scramble them over gentle heat. Avoid frying, as this raises AGE levels.							
Omelet							
w/butter	1 large		■				
w/cooking spray	1 large	■					
w/corn oil	1 large	■					
w/margarine	1 large	■					
w/olive oil	1 large	■					
Omelet, w/egg substitute	$^1/_4$ cup	■					
Poached	1 large	■					
Scrambled							
w/butter	1 large		■				
w/cooking spray	1 large	■					
w/corn oil	1 large	■					
w/margarine	1 large	■					
w/olive oil	1 large	■					

FOOD	Portion Size	Very Low 100 kU or less	Low 100–500 kU	Medium 501–1,000 kU	High 1,001–3,000 kU	Very High 3,001–5,000 kU	Highest 5,000–12,000 kU
			FAST FOODS				
Apple pie (McDonald's)	1 pie			■			
Bacon, egg & cheese biscuit	1 sandwich					■	
Cheeseburger	1 sandwich					■	
Cheeseburger, quarter-pound, double	1 sandwich						■
Chicken nuggets, fried	6 nuggets						■
Chicken sandwich							
crispy	1 sandwich						■
grilled	1 sandwich						■
Fish sandwich, fried	1 sandwich						■
French fries							
small	2.5 oz			■	■		
medium	4 oz				■		
large	6 oz				■	■	
Hamburger patty, beef	3 oz					■	
Hash brown potatoes	2 oz	■	■				
Hotcakes	3 hotcakes		■				

FOOD	Portion Size	Very Low 100 kU or less	Low 100–500 kU	Medium 501–1,000 kU	High 1,001–3,000 kU	Very High 3,001–5,000 kU	Highest 5,000–12,000 kU
FISH/SEAFOOD							
Crabmeat							
boiled	3 oz		■				
breaded, fried	3 oz					■	
Flounder							
oven-baked in parchment w/tomatoes	3 oz		■	■			
pan-cooked (nonstick), w/cooking spray	3 oz			■			
raw	3 oz		■				
Gefilte fish (fish loaf), boiled	3 oz			■			
Grouper							
grilled (nonstick grill), w/cooking spray	3 oz			■			
raw	3 oz		■				
Salmon, canned pink	3 oz			■			
Salmon fillet							
boiled	3 oz			■	■		
broiled	3 oz					■	
microwaved	3 oz			■			
pan-fried	3 oz				■	■	
poached	3 oz			■	■		
raw	3 oz		■				
smoked	3 oz			■			

FOOD	Portion Size	Very Low 100 kU or less	Low 100–500 kU	Medium 501–1,000 kU	High 1,001–3,000 kU	Very High 3,001–5,000 kU	Highest 5,000–12,000 kU
Scrod, broiled	3 oz		■	■			
Shrimp							
breaded, fried	3 oz					■	
marinated and barbecued	3 oz				■		
marinated w/lite balsamic dressing, broiled	3 oz			■			
raw	3 oz		■				
simmered in tomato/ white wine sauce	3 oz		■				
Trout							
baked	3 oz				■		
raw	3 oz			■			
Tuna							
baked	3 oz			■			
broiled w/vinaigrette	3 oz					■	
Tuna, canned							
chunk light in water	3 oz		■				
white albacore in oil	3 oz				■		
Tuna loaf, w/chunk light	3 oz			■			
Tuna patty, w/chunk light, broiled	3 oz			■			
Whiting, breaded, oven-fried	3 oz				■		
FRUIT							
Acai berries	3.5 oz	■					

FOOD	Portion Size	Very Low 100 kU or less	Low 100–500 kU	Medium 501–1,000 kU	High 1,001–3,000 kU	Very High 3,001–5,000 kU	Highest 5,000–12,000 kU
Apple							
baked	3.5 oz	■	■				
raw	3.5 oz	■					
simmered	3.5 oz	■					
Apricot							
baked	3.5 oz	■	■				
grilled	3.5 oz	■	■				
poached	3.5 oz	■					
raw	3.5 oz	■					
Avocado	1 oz		■				

TIP

Whenever possible, satisfy your sweet tooth with whole fresh fruit. It's low in AGEs and high in vitamins, minerals, and fiber.

FOOD	Portion Size	Very Low 100 kU or less	Low 100–500 kU	Medium 501–1,000 kU	High 1,001–3,000 kU	Very High 3,001–5,000 kU	Highest 5,000–12,000 kU
Banana							
baked	3.5 oz	■	■				
grilled	3.5 oz	■	■				
pan-fried w/cooking spray	3.5 oz	■	■				
raw	3.5 oz	■					
Blackberries							
cooked	3.5 oz	■					
raw	3.5 oz	■					
Blueberries							
cooked	3.5 oz	■					

FOOD	Portion Size	Very Low 100 kU or less	Low 100–500 kU	Medium 501–1,000 kU	High 1,001–3,000 kU	Very High 3,001–5,000 kU	Highest 5,000–12,000 kU
raw	3.5 oz	■					
Boysenberries							
cooked	3.5 oz	■					
raw	3.5 oz	■					
Cantaloupe							
grilled	3.5 oz	■	■				
raw	3.5 oz	■					
Cherries							
cooked	3.5 oz	■					
raw	3.5 oz	■					
Clementine	3.5 oz	■					
Cranberries							
cooked	3.5 oz	■					
raw	3.5 oz	■					
Crenshaw melon							
grilled	3.5 oz	■	■				
raw	3.5 oz	■					
Currants							
cooked	3.5 oz	■					
raw	3.5 oz	■					
Dates, chopped	1 oz	■					
Elderberries							
cooked	3.5 oz	■					
raw	3.5 oz	■					

FOOD	Portion Size	Very Low 100 kU or less	Low 100–500 kU	Medium 501–1,000 kU	High 1,001–3,000 kU	Very High 3,001–5,000 kU	Highest 5,000–12,000 kU
Fig, fresh							
grilled	3.5 oz	■	■				
raw	3.5 oz	■					
Goji berries	3.5 oz	■					
Grapefruit	3.5 oz	■					
Grapes							
cooked	3.5 oz	■					
raw	3.5 oz	■					
Honeydew melon							
grilled	3.5 oz	■	■				
raw	3.5 oz	■					
Huckleberries							
cooked	3.5 oz	■					
raw	3.5 oz	■					
Kiwifruit	3.5 oz	■					
Kumquat							
grilled	3.5 oz	■	■				
raw	3.5 oz	■					
roasted	3.5 oz	■	■				
Lemon	3.5 oz	■					
Lime	3.5 oz	■					
Loganberries							
cooked	3.5 oz	■					
raw	3.5 oz	■					

FOOD	Portion Size	Very Low 100 kU or less	Low 100–500 kU	Medium 501–1,000 kU	High 1,001–3,000 kU	Very High 3,001–5,000 kU	Highest 5,000–12,000 kU
Mango							
baked	3.5 oz						
grilled	3.5 oz						
raw	3.5 oz						
Mulberries							
cooked	3.5 oz						
raw	3.5 oz						
Nectarine							
baked	3.5 oz						
grilled	3.5 oz						
poached	3.5 oz						
raw	3.5 oz						
Orange	3.5 oz						
Papaya							
baked	3.5 oz						
grilled	3.5 oz						
raw	3.5 oz						
Passion fruit							
cooked	3.5 oz						
raw	3.5 oz						
Peach							
baked	3.5 oz						
grilled	3.5 oz						
poached	3.5 oz						

FOOD	Portion Size	Very Low 100 kU or less	Low 100–500 kU	Medium 501–1,000 kU	High 1,001–3,000 kU	Very High 3,001–5,000 kU	Highest 5,000–12,000 kU
raw	3.5 oz	■					
Pear							
baked	3.5 oz	■	■				
grilled	3.5 oz	■	■				
poached	3.5 oz	■					
raw	3.5 oz	■					
Persimmon							
cooked	3.5 oz	■					
raw	3.5 oz	■					
Pineapple							
baked	3.5 oz	■	■				
grilled	3.5 oz	■	■				
raw	3.5 oz	■					
Plantain							
baked	3.5 oz	■	■				
grilled	3.5 oz	■	■				
pan-cooked w/cooking spray	3.5 oz	■	■				
raw	3.5 oz	■					
Plum							
baked	3.5 oz	■	■				
grilled	3.5 oz	■	■				
poached	3.5 oz	■					
raw	3.5 oz	■					

FOOD	Portion Size	Very Low 100 kU or less	Low 100–500 kU	Medium 501–1,000 kU	High 1,001–3,000 kU	Very High 3,001–5,000 kU	Highest 5,000–12,000 kU
Pomegranate seeds	3.5 oz	■					
Prunes, pitted							
dried	1 oz	■					
stewed	1 oz	■					
Raisins							
cooked	1 oz	■					
dried	1 oz	■					
Raspberries							
cooked	3.5 oz	■					
raw	3.5 oz	■					
Star fruit	3.5 oz	■					
Strawberries							
cooked	3.5 oz	■					
raw	3.5 oz	■					
Tangerine	3.5 oz	■					
Watermelon							
grilled	3.5 oz	■	■				
raw	3.5 oz	■					
GRAINS							
Amaranth	3.5 oz	■					
Arborio rice	3.5 oz	■					
Barley	3.5 oz	■					
Basmati rice	3.5 oz	■					
Brown rice	3.5 oz	■					

FOOD	Portion Size	Very Low 100 kU or less	Low 100–500 kU	Medium 501–1,000 kU	High 1,001–3,000 kU	Very High 3,001–5,000 kU	Highest 5,000–12,000 kU
Buckwheat	3.5 oz	■					
Carnaroli rice	3.5 oz	■					
Carolina gold rice	3.5 oz	■					
Chinese black forbidden rice	3.5 oz	■					
Couscous	3.5 oz		■				
Emmer	3.5 oz	■					
Farro	3.5 oz	■					
Grits	3.5 oz	■					
Japonica rice, black	3.5 oz	■					
Jasmine rice	3.5 oz	■					
Kamut	3.5 oz	■					
Oats	3.5 oz	■					
Quinoa	3.5 oz	■					
Spelt	3.5 oz	■					
Wehani rice	3.5 oz	■					

TIP

Boiled and steamed whole grains such as brown rice, barley, farro, and quinoa are low in AGEs and high in fiber and nutrients, making them an important part of a healthy diet. To reduce carb and calorie counts, toss plenty of vegetables into your grain-based salads, side dishes, and casseroles.

White rice

FOOD	Portion Size	Very Low	Low	Medium	High	Very High	Highest
quick-cooking	3.5 oz	■					
regular	3.5 oz	■					

FOOD	Portion Size	Very Low 100 kU or less	Low 100–500 kU	Medium 501–1,000 kU	High 1,001–3,000 kU	Very High 3,001–5,000 kU	Highest 5,000–12,000 kU
Wild rice	3.5 oz	■					
			LAMB				
Lamb, from leg							
boiled	3 oz			■	■		
broiled	3 oz				■		
microwaved	3 oz			■	■		
raw	3 oz			■			

LEGUMES. ***See*** **Beans/Legumes.**

TIP

Although sausages that are fermented and air-dried (such as salami) and boiled meats (such as corned beef) appear to be relatively low in AGEs, they should be limited due to their high amounts of salt, nitrates, and other questionable ingredients. The regular consumption of processed meats has been linked to cancer.

LUNCHEON MEATS

FOOD	Portion Size	Very Low	Low	Medium	High	Very High	Highest
Bologna, beef	3 oz				■		
Frankfurter							
boiled	3 oz					■	■
broiled	3 oz						■
Ham, deli							
smoked	3 oz				■		
Virginia	3 oz			■			
Liverwurst	3 oz			■			
Salami, kosher	3 oz			■			

FOOD	Portion Size	Very Low 100 kU or less	Low 100–500 kU	Medium 501–1,000 kU	High 1,001–3,000 kU	Very High 3,001–5,000 kU	Highest 5,000–12,000 kU
MEAT. ***See*** **Beef/Beef Dishes; Lamb; Luncheon Meats; Pork/Pork Dishes.**							

TIP

A good way to fit ground beef into a low-AGE diet is to mix in chopped mushrooms. Meaty tasting and low in AGEs, mushrooms boost nutritional value and make meat portions go further. Replace up to a third of the meat in meatballs, burgers, and meatloaf, and up to half of the meat in tacos.

MUSHROOMS

FOOD	Portion Size	Very Low	Low	Medium	High	Very High	Highest
Baby bella (crimini)							
baked	3.5 oz	■	■				
boiled	3.5 oz	■					
broiled	3.5 oz	■	■				
grilled	3.5 oz	■	■				
raw	3.5 oz	■					
roasted	3.5 oz	■	■				
sautéed w/cooking spray	3.5 oz	■	■				
steamed	3.5 oz	■					
stir-fried w/cooking spray	3.5 oz	■	■				
Button (white button)							
baked	3.5 oz	■	■				
boiled	3.5 oz	■					
broiled	3.5 oz	■	■				
grilled	3.5 oz	■	■				
raw	3.5 oz	■					
roasted	3.5 oz	■	■				

FOOD	Portion Size	Very Low 100 kU or less	Low 100–500 kU	Medium 501–1,000 kU	High 1,001–3,000 kU	Very High 3,001–5,000 kU	Highest 5,000–12,000 kU
sautéed w/cooking spray	3.5 oz	■	■				
steamed	3.5 oz	■					
stir-fried w/cooking spray	3.5 oz	■	■				
Crimini. ***See*** **Baby bella.**							
Chanterelle							
baked	3.5 oz	■	■				
boiled	3.5 oz	■					
broiled	3.5 oz	■	■				
grilled	3.5 oz	■	■				
raw	3.5 oz	■					
roasted	3.5 oz	■	■				
sautéed w/cooking spray	3.5 oz	■	■				
steamed	3.5 oz	■					
stir-fried w/cooking spray	3.5 oz	■	■				
Enoki							
baked	3.5 oz	■	■				
boiled	3.5 oz	■					
broiled	3.5 oz	■	■				
grilled	3.5 oz	■	■				
raw	3.5 oz	■					
roasted	3.5 oz	■	■				
sautéed w/cooking spray	3.5 oz	■	■				
steamed	3.5 oz	■					
stir-fried w/cooking spray	3.5 oz	■	■				

FOOD	Portion Size	Very Low 100 kU or less	Low 100–500 kU	Medium 501–1,000 kU	High 1,001–3,000 kU	Very High 3,001–5,000 kU	Highest 5,000–12,000 kU
Morel							
baked	3.5 oz	■	■				
boiled	3.5 oz	■					
broiled	3.5 oz	■	■				
grilled	3.5 oz	■	■				
raw	3.5 oz	■					
roasted	3.5 oz	■	■				
sautéed w/cooking spray	3.5 oz	■	■				
steamed	3.5 oz	■					
stir-fried w/cooking spray	3.5 oz	■	■				
Oyster							
baked	3.5 oz	■	■				
boiled	3.5 oz	■					
broiled	3.5 oz	■	■				
grilled	3.5 oz	■	■				
raw	3.5 oz	■					
roasted	3.5 oz	■	■				
sautéed w/cooking spray	3.5 oz	■	■				
steamed	3.5 oz	■					
stir-fried w/cooking spray	3.5 oz	■	■				
Porcini							
baked	3.5 oz	■	■				
boiled	3.5 oz	■					
broiled	3.5 oz	■	■				

FOOD	Portion Size	Very Low 100 kU or less	Low 100–500 kU	Medium 501–1,000 kU	High 1,001–3,000 kU	Very High 3,001–5,000 kU	Highest 5,000–12,000 kU
grilled	3.5 oz	■	■				
raw	3.5 oz	■					
roasted	3.5 oz	■	■				
sautéed w/cooking spray	3.5 oz	■	■				
steamed	3.5 oz	■					
stir-fried w/cooking spray	3.5 oz	■	■				
Portobello							
baked	3.5 oz	■	■				
boiled	3.5 oz	■					
broiled	3.5 oz	■	■				
grilled	3.5 oz	■	■				
raw	3.5 oz	■					
roasted	3.5 oz	■	■				
sautéed w/cooking spray	3.5 oz	■	■				
steamed	3.5 oz	■					
stir-fried w/cooking spray	3.5 oz	■	■				
Shiitake							
baked	3.5 oz	■	■				
boiled	3.5 oz	■					
broiled	3.5 oz	■	■				
grilled	3.5 oz	■	■				
raw	3.5 oz	■					
roasted	3.5 oz	■	■				
sautéed w/cooking spray	3.5 oz	■	■				

FOOD	Portion Size	Very Low 100 kU or less	Low 100–500 kU	Medium 501–1,000 kU	High 1,001–3,000 kU	Very High 3,001–5,000 kU	Highest 5,000–12,000 kU
steamed	3.5 oz	■					
stir-fried w/cooking spray	3.5 oz	■	■				
Trumpet							
baked	3.5 oz	■	■				
boiled	3.5 oz	■					
broiled	3.5 oz	■	■				
grilled	3.5 oz	■	■				
raw	3.5 oz	■					
roasted	3.5 oz	■	■				
sautéed w/cooking spray	3.5 oz	■	■				
steamed	3.5 oz	■					
stir-fried w/cooking spray	3.5 oz	■	■				

White button. ***See* Button.**

TIP

Enjoy nuts in moderation—a one-ounce portion is reasonable—and choose raw nuts over roasted, as roasting increases AGE content. Although nuts are high in AGEs, they are a valuable addition to the diet because they provide fiber, protein, and other important nutrients.

NUTS/SEEDS

FOOD	Portion Size	Very Low	Low	Medium	High	Very High	Highest
Almonds							
raw	1 oz				■		
roasted	1 oz				■		
Cashews							
raw	1 oz				■		

FOOD	Portion Size	Very Low 100 kU or less	Low 100–500 kU	Medium 501–1,000 kU	High 1,001–3,000 kU	Very High 3,001–5,000 kU	Highest 5,000–12,000 kU
roasted	1 oz				■	■	
Chestnuts							
raw	1 oz			■			
roasted	1 oz				■		
Peanuts							
cocktail	1 oz				■		
dry roasted, unsalted	1 oz				■		
roasted in shell, salted	1 oz			■	■		
Pumpkin seeds, hulled, raw	1 oz			■			
Soybeans, roasted and salted	1 oz		■	■			
Sunflower seeds, hulled							
raw	1 oz			■			
roasted and salted	1 oz				■		
Walnuts, roasted	1 oz				■		
OIL							
Canola	1 Tbs			■			
Corn	1 Tbs				■		
Cottonseed	1 Tbs			■	■		

TIP

Keep in mind that when it comes to fats and oils, the AGE content can vary greatly. This variation depends on such factors as the product's age and whether it has been exposed to air, light, and/or heat—all of which increase oxidation and AGEs.

FOOD	Portion Size	Very Low 100 kU or less	Low 100–500 kU	Medium 501–1,000 kU	High 1,001–3,000 kU	Very High 3,001–5,000 kU	Highest 5,000–12,000 kU
Olive	1 Tbs		■				
Peanut	1 Tbs				■		
Safflower	1 Tbs		■	■			
Sesame	1 Tbs		■				
Sesame, toasted	1 Tbs					■	
Sunflower	1 Tbs			■			
PASTA/PASTA DISHES							
Couscous	3.5 oz		■				
Gnocchi, potato, w/parmesan cheese	3.5 oz			■			
Macaroni and cheese, baked	3.5 oz				■	■	
Pasta							
cooked al dente (7–8 minutes)	3.5 oz	■	■				
cooked well (11–12 minutes)	3.5 oz		■				
Pasta primavera	3.5 oz			■			
Pasta salad							
Italian	3.5 oz			■			
tuna	3.5 oz		■				
Ziti, baked	3.5 oz				■		
PORK/PORK DISHES							
Bacon							
microwaved	2 slices				■		

FOOD	Portion Size	Very Low 100 kU or less	Low 100–500 kU	Medium 501–1,000 kU	High 1,001–3,000 kU	Very High 3,001–5,000 kU	Highest 5,000–12,000 kU
pan-fried	2 slices						■
Ham, deli							
smoked	3 oz				■		
Virginia	3 oz			■			
Pork chop							
marinated w/vinegar, barbecued	3 oz				■	■	
marinated w/vinegar, raw	3 oz				■		
pan-fried	3 oz					■	
Ribs, roasted	3 oz					■	
Roast, loin							
oven-roasted	3 oz					■	
visibly lean, oven-braised w/beer	3 oz			■			
visibly lean, raw	3 oz		■				
Roast, tenderloin, lightly browned/braised	3 oz				■		
Sausage, Italian							
barbecued	3 oz					■	
raw	3 oz				■		
Sausage links							
beef and pork, pan-fried w/cooking spray	3 oz					■	■
pork, microwaved	3 oz					■	■

POULTRY. ***See* Chicken/Chicken Dishes; Turkey/Turkey Dishes.**

FOOD	Portion Size	Very Low 100 kU or less	Low 100–500 kU	Medium 501–1,000 kU	High 1,001–3,000 kU	Very High 3,001–5,000 kU	Highest 5,000–12,000 kU
SALAD DRESSINGS							
Blue cheese	1 Tbs	■	■				
Caesar	1 Tbs		■				
French	1 Tbs	■	■				
French, lite	1 Tbs	■					
Italian	1 Tbs	■	■				
Italian, lite	1 Tbs	■					
Thousand island	1 Tbs	■	■				
SAUCES. ***See*** **Dips/Spreads/Sauces.**							
SEAFOOD. ***See*** **Fish/Seafood.**							
SNACK FOODS. ***See also*** **Cakes/Pies/Baked Goods; Candy; Cookies/Crackers; Nuts/Seeds.**							
Breadsticks	1 oz	■					
Cheez Doodles, crunchy	1 oz			■			
Chex mix, traditional	1 oz		■				
Combos, nacho cheese pretzel	1 oz			■			
Corn chips	1 oz		■				
Fruit pop, frozen	2 oz	■					
Fruit roll-up	1 oz		■				
Gelatin, fruit-flavored							
regular	1/2 cup	■					
sugar-free	1/2 cup	■					

FOOD	Portion Size	Very Low 100 kU or less	Low 100–500 kU	Medium 501–1,000 kU	High 1,001–3,000 kU	Very High 3,001–5,000 kU	Highest 5,000–12,000 kU
Granola bar							
Chocolate Chunk (Quaker)	1 bar		■				
Peanut Butter/Chocolate Chip (Quaker)	1 bar			■			
Jerky, meatless	3 oz				■		
Nutrigrain Bar, Apple Cinnamon	1 bar			■			
Plantain chips	1 oz		■				
Pop tart							
microwaved	1 tart		■				
not heated	1 tart	■					
toasted	1 tart		■				
Popcorn							
air popped, w/butter	1 oz	■					
microwaved, fat-free	1 oz	■					
Potato chips							
baked	1 oz		■				
regular	1 oz			■			
Pretzels	1 oz		■	■			
Pudding, instant, all flavors							
fat-free, sugar-free	1/2 cup	■					
w/skim milk	1/2 cup	■					
Pudding, snack pack, all flavors	1/2 cup	■					

FOOD	Portion Size	Very Low 100 kU or less	Low 100–500 kU	Medium 501–1,000 kU	High 1,001–3,000 kU	Very High 3,001–5,000 kU	Highest 5,000–12,000 kU
Pumpkin seeds, hulled, raw	1 oz			■			
Rice cake, corn flavored	1 oz	■					
Rice Krispies Treat bar	1 bar		■	■			
Sorbet, fruit	$^{1}/_{2}$ cup	■					
Soybeans, roasted and salted	1 oz		■	■			
Sunflower seeds, hulled							
raw	1 oz			■			
roasted and salted	1 oz				■		
SOUPS							
Beef bouillon	1 cup	■					
Chicken bouillon	1 cup	■					
Chicken broth	1 cup	■					
Chicken noodle	1 cup	■					
Couscous and lentil	1 cup	■					
Cream of celery, low-fat	1 cup		■				
Lentil, vegetarian	1 cup		■				
Summer vegetable	1 cup	■					
Vegetable broth	1 cup	■					
SOY PRODUCTS							
Bacon bits, imitation (soy)	0.5 oz		■				
Boca Burger							
microwaved	1 burger	■					

FOOD	Portion Size	Very Low 100 kU or less	Low 100–500 kU	Medium 501–1,000 kU	High 1,001–3,000 kU	Very High 3,001–5,000 kU	Highest 5,000–12,000 kU
oven-baked	1 burger	■	■				
pan-cooked w/cooking spray	1 burger	■					
pan-cooked w/olive oil	1 burger		■				
Soymilk	1 cup	■					
Soy sauce	1 Tbs	■					
Soybeans, roasted and salted	1 oz		■	■			

TIP

Eat tofu raw, steamed, or simmered in soup. Broiling, grilling, or sautéing tofu causes a dramatic rise in AGEs.

FOOD	Portion Size	Very Low	Low	Medium	High	Very High	Highest
Tofu							
broiled	3 oz					■	
raw	3 oz			■			
sautéed	3 oz					■	
Tofu, soft							
boiled	3 oz			■			
raw	3 oz		■				
SPREADS. ***See* Dips/Spreads/Sauces.**							
SWEETENERS							
Aspartame, sugar substitute	1 tsp	■					
Caramel syrup, sugar-free	1 Tbs	■					
Corn syrup, dark	1 Tbs	■					
Dates, chopped	1 oz	■					

FOOD	Portion Size	Very Low 100 kU or less	Low 100–500 kU	Medium 501–1,000 kU	High 1,001–3,000 kU	Very High 3,001–5,000 kU	Highest 5,000–12,000 kU
Honey	1 Tbs	■					
Pancake syrup							
lite	1 Tbs	■					
regular	1 Tbs	■					
Sugar, granulated	1 tsp	■					
TURKEY/TURKEY DISHES							
Breast, skinless							
oven braised	3 oz			■	■		
raw	3 oz		■				
roasted	3 oz					■	
smoked, seared	3 oz						■
Burger							
broiled	3 oz					■	
pan-fried	3 oz						■
Burger, 94% lean							
pan-fried	3 oz				■		
Ground turkey							
grilled	3 oz						■
raw	3 oz					■	

TIP

Although sugar and high-sugar sweeteners are low in AGEs, their use should be limited. When sugar is added to foods and heated—when cookies are baked, for instance—the sugar can react with fats and proteins to make AGEs. Plus, a high-sugar diet can contribute to obesity, insulin resistance, and eventually, diabetes.

FOOD	Portion Size	Very Low 100 kU or less	Low 100–500 kU	Medium 501–1,000 kU	High 1,001–3,000 kU	Very High 3,001–5,000 kU	Highest 5,000–12,000 kU
Ground turkey, 94% lean							
pan-cooked w/cooking spray	3 oz			■	■		
raw	3 oz			■			
VEGETABLES. ***See also*** **Beans/Legumes; Mushrooms.**							
Acorn squash							
baked	3.5 oz	■	■				
boiled	3.5 oz	■					
broiled	3.5 oz	■	■				
grilled	3.5 oz	■	■				
raw	3.5 oz	■					
roasted	3.5 oz	■	■				
steamed	3.5 oz	■					
Arugula (rocket)	3.5 oz	■					
Asparagus							
boiled	3.5 oz	■					
broiled	3.5 oz	■	■				
grilled	3.5 oz	■	■				
raw	3.5 oz	■					
roasted	3.5 oz	■	■				
sautéed w/cooking spray	3.5 oz	■	■				
steamed	3.5 oz	■					
stir-fried w/cooking spray	3.5 oz	■	■				

FOOD	Portion Size	Very Low 100 kU or less	Low 100–500 kU	Medium 501–1,000 kU	High 1,001–3,000 kU	Very High 3,001–5,000 kU	Highest 5,000–12,000 kU
Aubergine. *See* Eggplant.							
Avocado	1 oz		■				
Beans, green. *See* Green beans.							
Beet (beetroot)							
boiled	3.5 oz	■					
raw	3.5 oz	■					
roasted	3.5 oz	■	■				
steamed	3.5 oz	■					
Beetroot. *See* Beet							
Belgian endive (endive, witloof)	3.5 oz	■					

TIP

To minimize AGE formation when sautéing vegetables, use a nonstick pan and either cooking spray or a small amount of olive oil—no more than a teaspoon per serving. This will help keep AGE counts in the "Low" or even the "Very Low" range. Using larger amounts of oil can drive the AGE count up to unhealthy levels.

FOOD	Portion Size	Very Low 100 kU or less	Low 100–500 kU	Medium 501–1,000 kU	High 1,001–3,000 kU	Very High 3,001–5,000 kU	Highest 5,000–12,000 kU
Bell pepper							
grilled	3.5 oz	■	■				
raw	3.5 oz	■					
roasted	3.5 oz	■	■				
sautéed w/cooking spray	3.5 oz	■	■				
steamed	3.5 oz	■					
stir-fried w/cooking spray	3.5 oz	■	■				

FOOD	Portion Size	Very Low 100 kU or less	Low 100–500 kU	Medium 501–1,000 kU	High 1,001–3,000 kU	Very High 3,001–5,000 kU	Highest 5,000–12,000 kU
Bibb lettuce	3.5 oz						
Bok choy							
boiled	3.5 oz						
broiled	3.5 oz						
grilled	3.5 oz						
raw	3.5 oz						
sautéed w/cooking spray	3.5 oz						
steamed	3.5 oz						
stir-fried w/cooking spray	3.5 oz						
Boston lettuce	3.5 oz						
Broccoli							
baked	3.5 oz						
boiled	3.5 oz						
broiled	3.5 oz						
grilled	3.5 oz						
raw	3.5 oz						
roasted	3.5 oz						
sautéed w/cooking spray	3.5 oz						
steamed	3.5 oz						
stir-fried w/cooking spray	3.5 oz						
Broccoli rabe (rapini)							
baked	3.5 oz						
boiled	3.5 oz						
raw	3.5 oz						

FOOD	Portion Size	Very Low 100 kU or less	Low 100–500 kU	Medium 501–1,000 kU	High 1,001–3,000 kU	Very High 3,001–5,000 kU	Highest 5,000–12,000 kU
sautéed w/cooking spray	3.5 oz	■	■				
steamed	3.5 oz	■					
stir-fried w/cooking spray	3.5 oz	■	■				
Broccolini							
baked	3.5 oz	■	■				
boiled	3.5 oz	■					
broiled	3.5 oz	■	■				
grilled	3.5 oz	■	■				
raw	3.5 oz	■					
roasted	3.5 oz	■	■				
sautéed w/cooking spray	3.5 oz	■	■				
steamed	3.5 oz	■					
stir-fried w/cooking spray	3.5 oz	■	■				

TIP

Vegetables are naturally low in AGEs because of their relatively low content of protein and fat and their high content of water. Grilling, broiling, and roasting can increase their AGE content —especially when butter or oil are used—but even when prepared using these methods, veggies still have just a minute fraction of the AGEs found in grilled and broiled meats.

FOOD	Portion Size	Very Low 100 kU or less	Low 100–500 kU	Medium 501–1,000 kU	High 1,001–3,000 kU	Very High 3,001–5,000 kU	Highest 5,000–12,000 kU
Brussels sprouts							
baked	3.5 oz	■	■				
boiled	3.5 oz	■					
broiled	3.5 oz	■	■				
grilled	3.5 oz	■	■				

FOOD	Portion Size	Very Low 100 kU or less	Low 100– 500 kU	Medium 501– 1,000 kU	High 1,001– 3,000 kU	Very High 3,001– 5,000 kU	Highest 5,000– 12,000 kU
raw	3.5 oz	■					
roasted	3.5 oz	■	■				
sautéed w/cooking spray	3.5 oz	■	■				
steamed	3.5 oz	■					
stir-fried w/cooking spray	3.5 oz	■	■				
Butter lettuce	3.5 oz	■					
Butternut squash							
baked	3.5 oz	■	■				
boiled	3.5 oz	■					
broiled	3.5 oz	■	■				
grilled	3.5 oz	■	■				
raw	3.5 oz	■					
roasted	3.5 oz	■	■				
steamed	3.5 oz	■					
Cabbage							
boiled	3.5 oz	■					
raw	3.5 oz	■					
sautéed w/cooking spray	3.5 oz	■	■				
steamed	3.5 oz	■					
stir-fried w/cooking spray	3.5 oz	■	■				
Carrots							
baked	3.5 oz	■	■				
boiled	3.5 oz	■					
broiled	3.5 oz	■	■				

FOOD	Portion Size	Very Low 100 kU or less	Low 100–500 kU	Medium 501–1,000 kU	High 1,001–3,000 kU	Very High 3,001–5,000 kU	Highest 5,000–12,000 kU
canned, unheated	3.5 oz	■					
grilled	3.5 oz	■	■				
raw	3.5 oz	■					
roasted	3.5 oz	■	■				
sautéed w/cooking spray	3.5 oz	■	■				
steamed	3.5 oz	■					
stir-fried w/cooking spray	3.5 oz	■	■				
Cauliflower							
baked	3.5 oz	■	■				
boiled	3.5 oz	■					
broiled	3.5 oz	■	■				
grilled	3.5 oz	■	■				
raw	3.5 oz	■					
roasted	3.5 oz	■	■				
sautéed w/cooking spray	3.5 oz	■	■				
steamed	3.5 oz	■					
stir-fried w/cooking spray	3.5 oz	■	■				
Celery							
boiled	3.5 oz	■					
broiled	3.5 oz	■	■				
grilled	3.5 oz	■	■				
raw	3.5 oz	■					
roasted	3.5 oz	■	■				
steamed	3.5 oz	■					

FOOD	Portion Size	Very Low 100 kU or less	Low 100–500 kU	Medium 501–1,000 kU	High 1,001–3,000 kU	Very High 3,001–5,000 kU	Highest 5,000–12,000 kU
stir-fried w/cooking spray	3.5 oz	■	■				
Chard. *See* Swiss chard.							
Chicory (curly endive, frisee)	3.5 oz	■					
Collard greens							
baked	3.5 oz	■	■				
boiled	3.5 oz	■					
raw	3.5 oz	■					
sautéed w/cooking spray	3.5 oz	■	■				
steamed	3.5 oz	■					
stir-fried w/cooking spray	3.5 oz	■	■				

TIP

Keep the amount of AGEs in vegetables low by going easy on added fats. A good tip is to add just a drizzle of extra-virgin olive oil instead of drenching your dish with oil, butter, or cheese sauce.

FOOD	Portion Size	Very Low 100 kU or less	Low 100–500 kU	Medium 501–1,000 kU	High 1,001–3,000 kU	Very High 3,001–5,000 kU	Highest 5,000–12,000 kU
Corn							
baked	3.5 oz	■	■				
boiled	3.5 oz	■					
broiled	3.5 oz	■	■				
canned, unheated	3.5 oz	■					
grilled	3.5 oz	■	■				
microwaved	3.5 oz	■					
raw	3.5 oz	■					

FOOD	Portion Size	Very Low 100 kU or less	Low 100–500 kU	Medium 501–1,000 kU	High 1,001–3,000 kU	Very High 3,001–5,000 kU	Highest 5,000–12,000 kU
roasted	3.5 oz	■	■				
sautéed w/cooking spray	3.5 oz	■	■				
steamed	3.5 oz	■					
stir-fried w/cooking spray	3.5 oz	■	■				
Cos lettuce. *See* Romaine lettuce.							
Courgette. *See* Zucchini.							
Cress. *See* Watercress.							
Cucumber							
baked	3.5 oz	■	■				
grilled	3.5 oz	■	■				
raw	3.5 oz	■					
roasted	3.5 oz	■	■				
stir-fried w/cooking spray	3.5 oz	■	■				
Curly endive. *See* Chicory.							
Dandelion greens							
boiled	3.5 oz	■					
raw	3.5 oz	■					
sautéed w/cooking spray	3.5 oz	■	■				
steamed	3.5 oz	■					
stir-fried w/cooking spray	3.5 oz	■	■				
Eggplant (aubergine)							
broiled	3.5 oz	■	■				
grilled	3.5 oz	■	■				

FOOD	Portion Size	Very Low 100 kU or less	Low 100–500 kU	Medium 501–1,000 kU	High 1,001–3,000 kU	Very High 3,001–5,000 kU	Highest 5,000–12,000 kU
raw	3.5 oz	■					
roasted	3.5 oz	■	■				
sautéed w/cooking spray	3.5 oz	■	■				
steamed	3.5 oz	■					
stewed	3.5 oz	■					
stir-fried w/cooking spray	3.5 oz	■	■				
Endive. ***See*** **Belgian endive.**							
Escarole							
boiled	3.5 oz	■					
raw	3.5 oz	■					
sautéed w/cooking spray	3.5 oz	■	■				
steamed							
stir-fried w/cooking spray	3.5 oz	■	■				
Frisee. ***See*** **Chicory.**							
Garlic							
raw	1 oz	■					
roasted	1 oz	■	■				
sautéed w/cooking spray	1 oz	■	■				
stir-fried w/cooking spray	1 oz	■	■				
Green beans							
baked	3.5 oz	■	■				
boiled	3.5 oz	■					
canned, unheated	3.5 oz	■					
raw	3.5 oz	■					

FOOD	Portion Size	Very Low 100 kU or less	Low 100–500 kU	Medium 501–1,000 kU	High 1,001–3,000 kU	Very High 3,001–5,000 kU	Highest 5,000–12,000 kU
sautéed w/cooking spray	3.5 oz	■	■				
steamed	3.5 oz	■					
stir-fried w/cooking spray	3.5 oz	■	■				
Green onion (scallion)							
boiled	3.5 oz	■					
broiled	3.5 oz	■	■				
grilled	3.5 oz	■	■				
raw	3.5 oz	■					
roasted	3.5 oz	■	■				
sautéed w/cooking spray	3.5 oz	■	■				
steamed	3.5 oz	■					
stir-fried w/cooking spray	3.5 oz	■	■				
Iceberg lettuce	3.5 oz	■					
Jicama							
baked	3.5 oz	■	■				
boiled	3.5 oz	■					
raw	3.5 oz	■					
roasted	3.5 oz	■	■				
sautéed w/cooking spray	3.5 oz	■	■				
steamed	3.5 oz	■					
stir-fried w/cooking spray	3.5 oz	■	■				
Kale							
baked	3.5 oz	■	■				
boiled	3.5 oz	■					

FOOD	Portion Size	Very Low 100 kU or less	Low 100–500 kU	Medium 501–1,000 kU	High 1,001–3,000 kU	Very High 3,001–5,000 kU	Highest 5,000–12,000 kU
raw	3.5 oz	■					
roasted	3.5 oz	■	■				
sautéed w/cooking spray	3.5 oz	■	■				
steamed	3.5 oz	■					
Leeks							
baked	3.5 oz	■	■				
boiled	3.5 oz	■					
broiled	3.5 oz	■	■				
grilled	3.5 oz	■	■				
raw	3.5 oz	■					
roasted	3.5 oz	■	■				
sautéed w/cooking spray	3.5 oz	■	■				
steamed	3.5 oz	■					
stir-fried w/cooking spray	3.5 oz	■	■				
Mache salad greens	3.5 oz	■					
Mizuna salad greens	3.5 oz	■					
Mustard greens							
boiled	3.5 oz	■					
raw	3.5 oz	■					
sautéed w/cooking spray	3.5 oz	■	■				
steamed	3.5 oz	■					
stir-fried w/cooking spray	3.5 oz	■	■				
Okra							
boiled	3.5 oz	■					

FOOD	Portion Size	Very Low 100 kU or less	Low 100–500 kU	Medium 501–1,000 kU	High 1,001–3,000 kU	Very High 3,001–5,000 kU	Highest 5,000–12,000 kU
broiled	3.5 oz						
grilled	3.5 oz						
roasted	3.5 oz						
steamed	3.5 oz						
Onion							
baked	3.5 oz						
boiled	3.5 oz						
broiled	3.5 oz						
grilled	3.5 oz						
raw	3.5 oz						
roasted	3.5 oz						
sautéed w/cooking spray	3.5 oz						
steamed	3.5 oz						
stir-fried w/cooking spray	3.5 oz						
Parsnip							
baked	3.5 oz						
boiled	3.5 oz						
raw	3.5 oz						
roasted	3.5 oz						
sautéed w/cooking spray	3.5 oz						
steamed	3.5 oz						
stir-fried w/cooking spray	3.5 oz						
Potato, sweet							
baked	3.5 oz						

FOOD	Portion Size	Very Low 100 kU or less	Low 100–500 kU	Medium 501–1,000 kU	High 1,001–3,000 kU	Very High 3,001–5,000 kU	Highest 5,000–12,000 kU
boiled	3.5 oz	■					
roasted	3.5 oz	■	■				
steamed	3.5 oz	■					
Potato, white							
baked	3.5 oz	■	■				
boiled	3.5 oz	■					
roasted	3.5 oz	■	■				
steamed	3.5 oz	■					
Pumpkin							
baked	3.5 oz	■	■				
boiled	3.5 oz	■					
raw	3.5 oz	■					
roasted	3.5 oz	■	■				
sautéed w/cooking spray	3.5 oz	■	■				
steamed	3.5 oz	■					
Radicchio	3.5 oz	■					
Radish							
grilled	3.5 oz	■	■				
raw	3.5 oz	■					
roasted	3.5 oz	■	■				
Ramps (wild leeks)							
baked	3.5 oz	■	■				
boiled	3.5 oz	■					
broiled	3.5 oz	■	■				

FOOD	Portion Size	Very Low 100 kU or less	Low 100–500 kU	Medium 501–1,000 kU	High 1,001–3,000 kU	Very High 3,001–5,000 kU	Highest 5,000–12,000 kU
grilled	3.5 oz	■	■				
raw	3.5 oz	■					
roasted	3.5 oz	■	■				
sautéed w/cooking spray	3.5 oz	■	■				
steamed	3.5 oz	■					
stir-fried w/cooking spray	3.5 oz	■	■				
Rapini. ***See*** **Broccoli rabe.**							
Rocket. ***See*** **Arugula.**							
Romaine lettuce (cos)	3.5 oz	■					
Rutabaga (swede)							
baked	3.5 oz	■	■				
boiled	3.5 oz	■					
braised	3.5 oz	■					
raw	3.5 oz	■					
roasted	3.5 oz	■	■				
sautéed w/cooking spray	3.5 oz	■	■				
steamed	3.5 oz	■					
stir-fried w/cooking spray	3.5 oz	■	■				
Scallion. ***See*** **Green onion.**							
Spaghetti squash							
baked	3.5 oz	■	■				
boiled	3.5 oz	■					
roasted	3.5 oz	■	■				
sautéed w/cooking spray	3.5 oz	■	■				

FOOD	Portion Size	Very Low 100 kU or less	Low 100–500 kU	Medium 501–1,000 kU	High 1,001–3,000 kU	Very High 3,001–5,000 kU	Highest 5,000–12,000 kU
steamed	3.5 oz	■					
Spinach							
boiled	3.5 oz	■					
raw	3.5 oz	■					
sautéed w/cooking spray	3.5 oz	■	■				
steamed	3.5 oz	■					
stir-fried w/cooking spray	3.5 oz	■	■				
Swede. ***See*** **Rutabaga.**							
Sweet potato. ***See*** **Potato, sweet.**							
Swiss chard							
boiled	3.5 oz	■					
raw	3.5 oz	■					
sautéed w/cooking spray	3.5 oz	■	■				
steamed	3.5 oz	■					
stir-fried w/cooking spray	3.5 oz	■	■				
Tatsoi salad greens	3.5 oz	■					
Tomato							
baked	3.5 oz	■	■				
boiled	3.5 oz	■					
broiled	3.5 oz	■	■				
grilled	3.5 oz	■	■				
raw	3.5 oz	■					
roasted	3.5 oz	■	■				
steamed	3.5 oz	■					

FOOD	Portion Size	Very Low 100 kU or less	Low 100–500 kU	Medium 501–1,000 kU	High 1,001–3,000 kU	Very High 3,001–5,000 kU	Highest 5,000–12,000 kU
Turnip							
baked	3.5 oz	■	■				
boiled	3.5 oz	■					
raw	3.5 oz	■					
roasted	3.5 oz	■	■				
sautéed w/cooking spray	3.5 oz	■	■				
steamed	3.5 oz	■					
stir-fried w/cooking spray	3.5 oz	■	■				
Watercress (cress)	3.5 oz	■					
Wild leeks. *See* Ramps.							
Witloof. *See* Belgian endive.							
Zucchini (courgette)							
baked	3.5 oz	■	■				
boiled	3.5 oz	■					
broiled	3.5 oz	■	■				
grilled	3.5 oz	■	■				
raw	3.5 oz	■					
roasted	3.5 oz	■	■				
sautéed w/cooking spray	3.5 oz	■	■				
steamed	3.5 oz	■					
stir-fried w/cooking spray	3.5 oz	■	■				

INDEX

OTHER SQUAREONE TITLES OF INTEREST

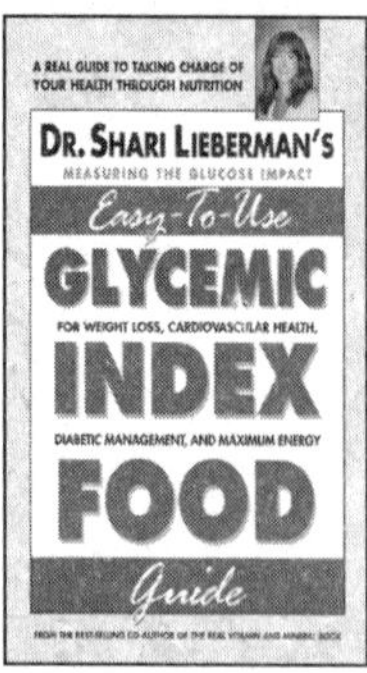

GLYCEMIC INDEX FOOD GUIDE

For Weight Loss, Cardiovascular Health, Diabetic Management, and Maximum Energy

Dr. Shari Lieberman

By indicating how quickly a given food causes a rise in blood sugar, the glycemic index (GI) enables you to choose foods that can help you manage a variety of conditions and improve your overall health. This easy-to-use guide teaches you about the GI and how to use it. It provides both the glycemic index and the glycemic load for hundreds of foods and beverages. Whether you want to manage your diabetes, lose weight, increase your heart health, or simply enhance your well-being, the *Glycemic Index Food Guide* is the best place to start.

$7.95 • 160 pages • 4 x 7-inch paperback • ISBN 978-0-7570-0245-8

THE ACID-ALKALINE FOOD GUIDE, SECOND EDITION

A Quick Reference to Foods & Their Effect on pH Levels

Susan E. Brown, PhD, and Larry Trivieri, Jr.

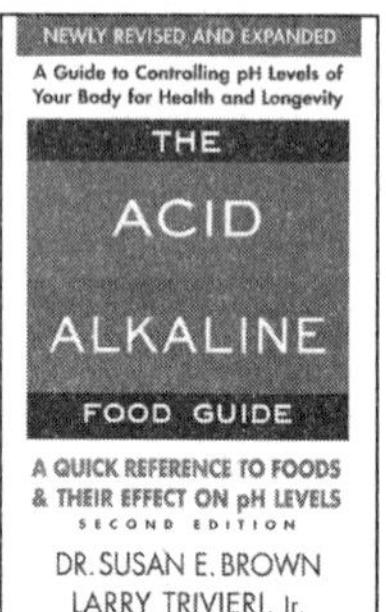

The importance of acid-alkaline balance to good health is no secret. *The Acid-Alkaline Food Guide* was designed as an easy-to-follow guide to the most common foods that influence your body's pH level. Now in its Second Edition, this bestseller has been expanded to include many more domestic and international foods. Updated information also explores (and refutes) the myths about pH balance and diet, and guides you to supplements that can help you achieve a pH level that supports greater well-being.

$8.95 • 224 pages • 4 x 7-inch paperback • ISBN 978-0-7570-0393-6

Dr. Vlassara's A.G.E.-Less Diet

How Chemicals in the Foods We Eat Promote Disease, Obesity, and Aging And the Steps We Can Take to Stop It

Helen Vlassara, MD, Sandra Woodruff, MS, RD, and Gary E. Striker, MD

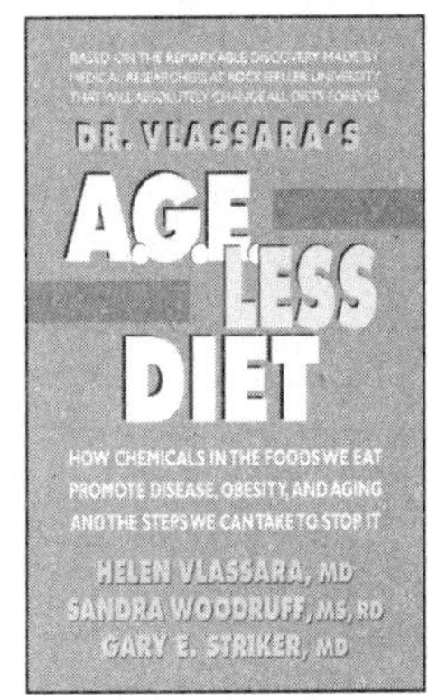

Imagine naturally occurring toxins that are directly responsible for inflammation, chronic diseases, and aging. While that may not have been what Dr. Helen Vlassara was looking for when she began her work at the research laboratories of Rockefeller University, it was what her pioneering team discovered in 1985. Trying to understand why patients with diabetes were prone to develop heart, eye, kidney, nerve, and circulatory disorders, as well as other signs of premature aging, the team focused on compounds called *advanced glycation end products,* or *AGEs.*

Dr. Vlassara's research revealed that AGEs enter the body through the digestive tract via the diet, and that there is a tremendous difference between an AGE-laden diet and an AGE-less diet. AGEs simply accelerate the body's aging process by increasing oxidation and free radicals, hardening tissue, and creating chronic inflammation.

For years, these amazing studies have remained relatively unknown to the public and even the medical community. Now, Dr. Helen Vlassara and best-selling author Sandra Woodruff have written a complete guide to understanding what AGEs are and how you can avoid them through the careful selection of foods and cooking techniques. In *Dr. Vlassara's AGE-Less Diet,* the authors offer simple principles that can be applied to your diet—or to any popular diet—to lower your intake of AGEs. They include an AGE ranking of foods as well as recipes that reduce your consumption of AGEs.

By lowering your AGE levels, you can reduce the potential of developing any number of serious disorders, look years younger, and enjoy greater health and longevity. *Dr. Vlassara's AGE-Less Diet* guides you in making a real and important difference in your life.

$16.95 US • 328 pages • 6 x 9-inch paperback • ISBN 978-0-7570-0420-9

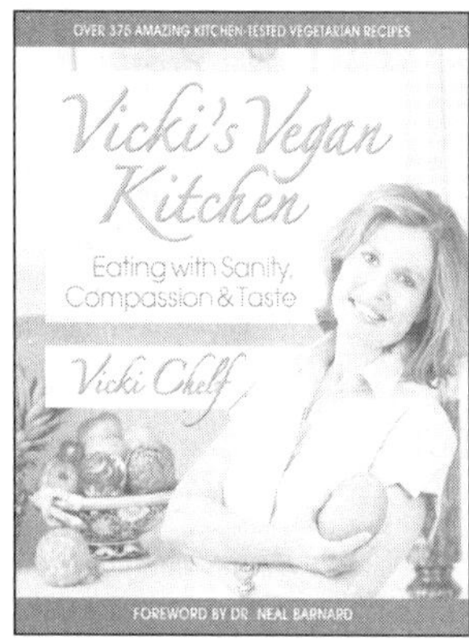

Vicki's Vegan Kitchen

Eating with Sanity, Compassion & Taste

Vicki Chelf

Vegan dishes are healthy, delicious, and surprisingly easy to make. Yet many people are daunted by the idea of preparing meals that contain no animal products. For them, and for everyone who loves great food, vegetarian chef Vicki Chelf presents *Vicki's Vegan Kitchen,* a comprehensive cookbook designed to take the mysteryout of meatless meals.

The book begins with an overview of the vegan diet, including its nutritional benefits and impact on weight control. Chapters on kitchen staples, cooking methods, and food preparation techniques come next, along with helpful guidelines on shopping for the best-quality foods and ingredients. Over 375 of Vicki's favorite recipes and recipe variations follow. She shares delectable breakfast choices—from pancakes and waffles to hot cereals and scrambles—and shows you how to make to make heavenly breads, perfect pie crusts, and incredible homemade pasta (you won't believe how easy it is). You'll even learn how to make your own "moo-less" milks! Vicki also provides her collection of luscious dips and spreads, sensational soups and salads, satisfying bean dishes; pilafs and other grain creations; veggie favorites; a collection of scrumptious desserts; and so much more. To help ensure successful results, step-by-step directions accompany each recipe, and instructional drawings appear throughout. Every dish is a winner—easy to make, completely vegan, and utterly delicious.

Whether you're interested in compassionate cooking, you value the benefits of a meat-free diet, or you just want to treat your family to a wonderful meal, *Vicki's Vegan Kitchen* will bring delectable vegan fare to your kitchen table.

$17.95 US • 320 pages • 7.5 x 9-inch paperback • ISBN 978-0-7570-0251-9

The Change Cookbook

Using the Power of Food to Transform Your Body, Your Health, and Your Life

Milan Ross and Scott Stoll, MD

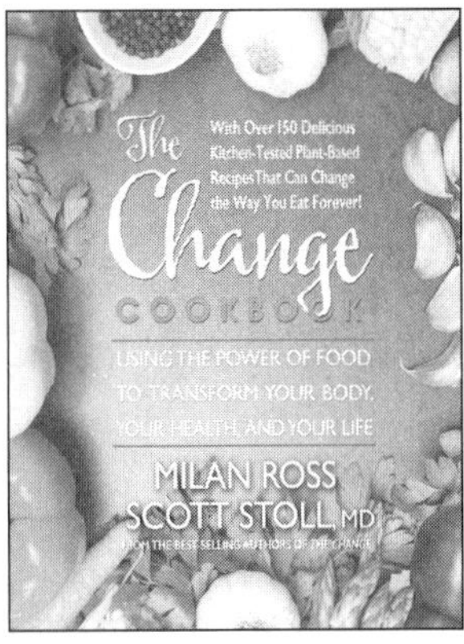

From the best-selling authors of *The Change* comes a new cookbook based on Dr. Stoll's Immersion program for weight loss and better health. Imagine dishes that can reduce your cholesterol, lower your blood pressure, boost your immune system, and decrease your odds of getting cancer, type 2 diabetes, heart disease, strokes, and a host of other all-too-common health problems. Here, in this new book, are over 150 recipes that can truly change your life for the better.

Part One begins with the journey taken by each author to develop such a cookbook. This section shares the plant-based food principles that have propelled their book *The Change* to become a bestseller. This is followed by an overview of a plant-based diet, including its nutritional benefits and impact on weight control. Subsequent chapters provide important information on kitchen staples, cooking methods, food preparation techniques, and helpful guidelines on shopping for the best-quality foods and ingredients.

In Part Two, the authors share over 150 kitchen-tested recipes for delectable dishes. Included are satisfying breakfast choices, luscious dips and spreads, sensational soups and salads, satisfying bean dishes, hearty pilafs and other grain creations, and veggie favorites, topped off with a collection of fantastic desserts. Each recipe provides easy-to-follow directions that ensure success.

$17.95 US • 256 pages • 7.5 x 9-inch paperback • ISBN 978-0-7570-0438-4

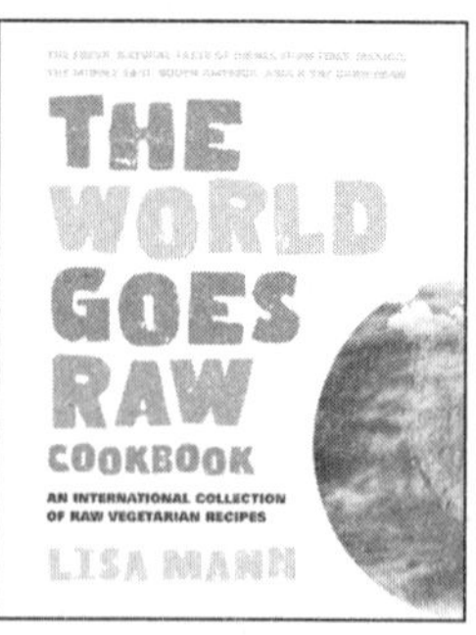

The World Goes Raw Cookbook

An International Collection of Raw Vegetarian Recipes

Lisa Mann

Although raw food can be delicious and improve your well-being, raw cuisine cookbooks have always offered little variety—until now. In *The World Goes Raw Cookbook,* chef Lisa Mann provides a fresh approach to (un)cooking. Lisa first guides you in stocking your kitchen and then presents six chapters of international dishes, including Italian, Mexican, Middle Eastern, Asian, Caribbean, and South American cuisine. Let *The World Goes Raw* add variety to your life while helping you feel healthier and more energized than ever before.

$16.95 US • 176 pages • 7.5 x 9-inch paperback • ISBN 978-0-7570-0320-2

Eat Smart, Eat Raw

Creative Vegetarian Recipes for a Healthier Life

Kate Wood

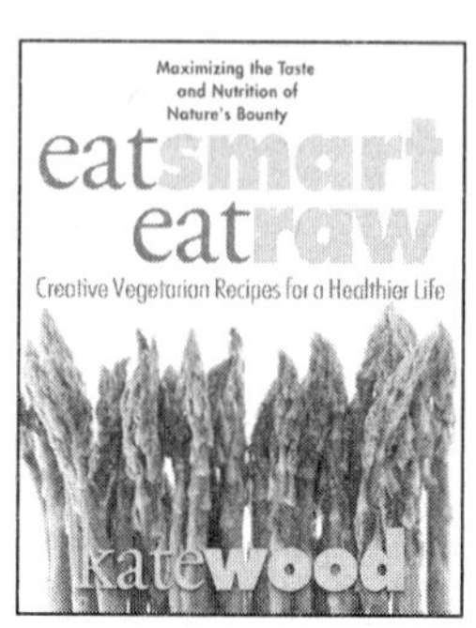

As the popularity of raw vegetarian cuisine soars, so does the evidence that uncooked food is amazingly good for you. Now there is another reason to go raw—taste! In *Eat Smart, Eat Raw,* Kate Wood presents 150 recipes for truly exceptional dishes, including hearty breakfasts, savory soups, satisfying entrées, and luscious desserts. Whether you are an ardent vegetarian or just someone in search of a great meal, this book may forever change the way you look at an oven.

$15.95 US • 184 pages • 7.5 x 9-inch paperback • ISBN 978-0-7570-0261-8